Natural Beauties

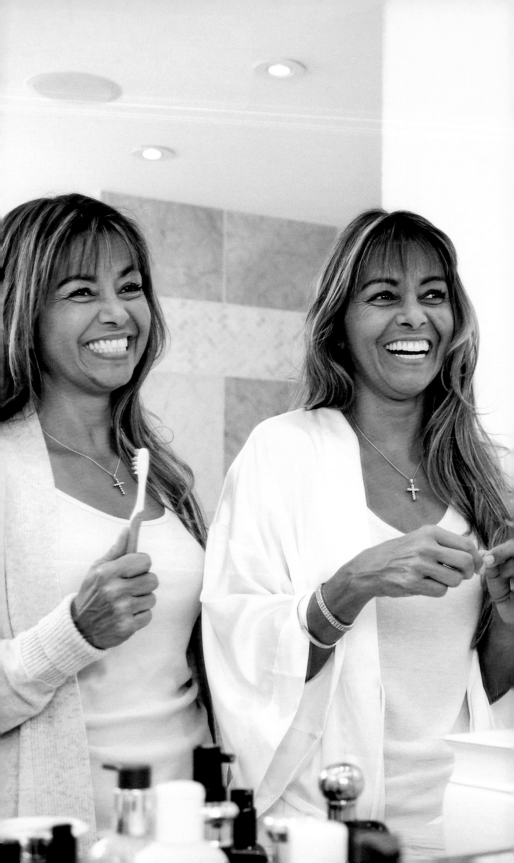

MARITA AND MIMINA MEZA

Natural Beauties

HOMEMADE WELLNESS TIPS
from Head to Toe

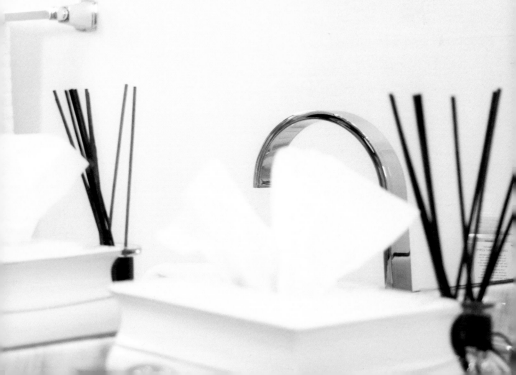

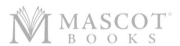

www.mascotbooks.com

Natural Beauties: Homemade Wellness Tips from Head to Toe

An important note: All the information in this book is to help inform you of natural solutions for your health and beauty. The advice and recommendations do not substitute a medical consultation, or serve as professional medical advice.

For more information, please contact:
Mascot Books
620 Herndon Parkway, Suite 320
Herndon, VA 20170
info@mascotbooks.com

Library of Congress Control Number: 2021905228

CPSIA Code: PRFRE0621A
ISBN-13: 978-1-64543-703-1

Printed in Canada

Contents

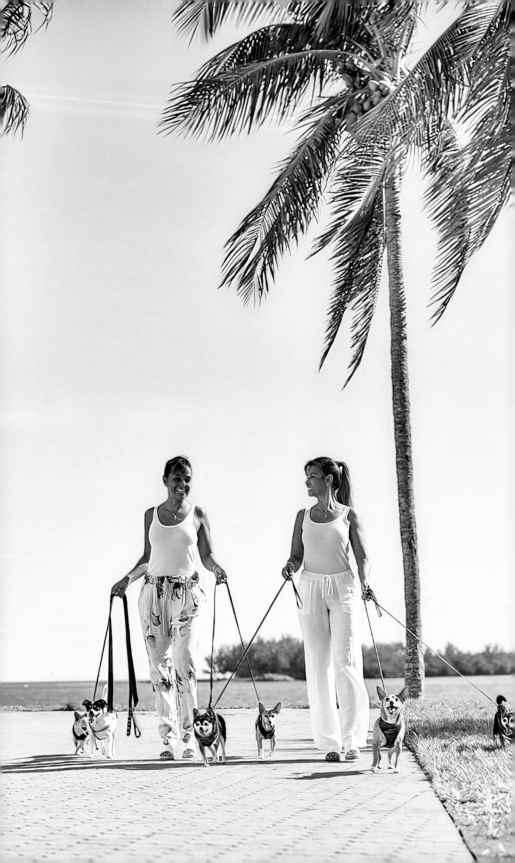

Introduction

As identical twin sisters, we have always been best friends. We grew up in a small town in Venezuela, where everyone had a hard time telling us apart. When we were four years old, we started performing, both dancing and acting, because we loved being the center of attention. We would dress alike, style our hair the same way, and soak in the attention!

We were also very mischievous and used our identical appearances to our advantage, switching places whenever it suited us. No one knew when we went to each other's classes or traded places in after-school activities. It was great fun!

But as we got older, certain things became dead giveaways for others to tell us apart. Neither of us wanted to be the sister you could recognize by her pimples, chipped manicure, split ends, or plumper frame. So, to maintain our identical looks, we took incredibly good care of ourselves. Our mother and grandmother had many time-tested beauty rituals and secrets, and we grew up watching and emulating them.

When we were twelve, we started modeling and competing in beauty pageants, acts that played a significant role in our commitment to beauty and fitness from a young age. Whenever companies wanted to book twins around our age, we nearly always got the job—on top of sports, activities, and of course our academics. We were busy!

It was easy to see how beauty was opening doors for us. After high school, we were able to leave our small town and travel the world, getting paid for work we enjoyed. Marita became somewhat of a sensation in the pageant world. She participated in the contest for Miss Clin d'oeil Magazine, won Miss Pava 1982 and Miss Beautiful in 1982, Miss Merida, Top Model of the Year in Merida, Miss Caribbean Queen in Montreal, and even the second runner-up in the national Miss Hawaiian Tropic pageant in Canada! The lifestyle was like something out of a dream. There were amazing parties, glamorous clothes, and carefree living.

It was also incredibly hard work. We routinely worked sixteen-hour days, and we were exhausted. We would wake up early for a photo shoot, then come home and want nothing more than to lie down. But we needed to squeeze in a workout and make a healthy dinner before working another job in the evening. Many evening bookings were events, where people would be partying. Our mouths watered as our clients and friends devoured delicious hors d'oeuvres and indulged in bottomless champagne, eating and drinking whatever they pleased. We were almost always on a very strict diet to maintain our physique, and it was hard to stay disciplined! After getting home late at night, instead of falling into our beds with our makeup still on, we had to prepare for another early-morning shoot, where we were expected to look fresh-faced and beautiful. The lifestyle was both fun and exhausting.

Over the years, we learned a ton about taking care of our skin, hair, nails, and teeth. We learned how to eat properly, exercise right, get our vitamins, and stay active and healthy. We also learned tips and tricks for using affordable, natural ingredients as beauty and wellness products. We put them to the test for ourselves, creating masks, creams, and scrubs. If the recipes didn't make a real difference, we moved on to something else.

Though our careers are outside of modeling now—Mimina works in hospitality and Marita in the family foundation Fundación Solidarios con Venezuela—we still take care of ourselves and our appearance. It feels good to be fit, healthy, and looking younger than we really are! We've learned that self-care really isn't that hard. Instead of making it an indulgence when we find the time, we do a little every day to focus on ourselves. We hope you will prioritize yourself in the same way! That is a key reason why we are writing this book. There are too many women who put themselves last—after their kids, significant other, job, family, and friends. They think they don't have enough time or money to take care of themselves, but that just isn't true. We want to show women how taking care of yourself doesn't mean compromising other parts of your life. It is easy to look twenty years younger and more beautiful, and simple changes that make a noticeable difference can easily fit into your life.

This book contains only the best beauty advice and recipes from our many years of modeling and pageants, and it's all rooted in natural ingredients. We believe nature provides everything you need for a beauty regimen that will keep you looking younger while staying healthy. Of course, there are many products you can buy, but these products are created from essentially two groups of ingredients: natural products from the earth and chemicals. It's smart to avoid chemicals because many of them are linked to cancer, reproductive issues, and other illnesses (yes, you read that right). Many products that are legally sold and well-loved by consumers contain harmful ingredients. The industry should be better regulated so that doesn't happen, but the reality is that many commercial beauty products just aren't safe. They might contain powerful natural ingredients like aloe, green tea, honey, or coconut oil, but they're mixed with things you don't want in or on your body. And unfortunately, chemicals are usually introduced to consumers long before proper testing has determined whether those ingredients pose health risks. That chemicals aren't on "the naughty list" yet doesn't mean they won't ultimately be added to it. Remember: there was a time asbestos insulated our homes, lead was a key ingredient in paint, and cigarettes were marketed as healthy. By the time the government makes harmful chemicals illegal, it's often too late for the people who have been exposed to them regularly over the years. Beauty products are no different, except for the fact that your exposure to them is even more intimate. When you rub products onto your skin, the chemicals are absorbed directly into your body, both through your skin and inhalation (fragrance itself often contains harmful ingredients and is a totally unnecessary aspect of beauty products). When you take a chance on beauty products without doing your research, you're putting yourself at risk.

This is a huge reason why we believe in using simple, natural ingredients. Instead of searching for beauty products that don't contain harmful chemicals, it's easier and less expensive to make your own products at home. In this book, we will show you how. We've been using these recipes for years, and we can tell you that they work wonders! People almost always assume we are much younger than we are because our beauty secrets are so good! We can't wait to share them with you in this book.

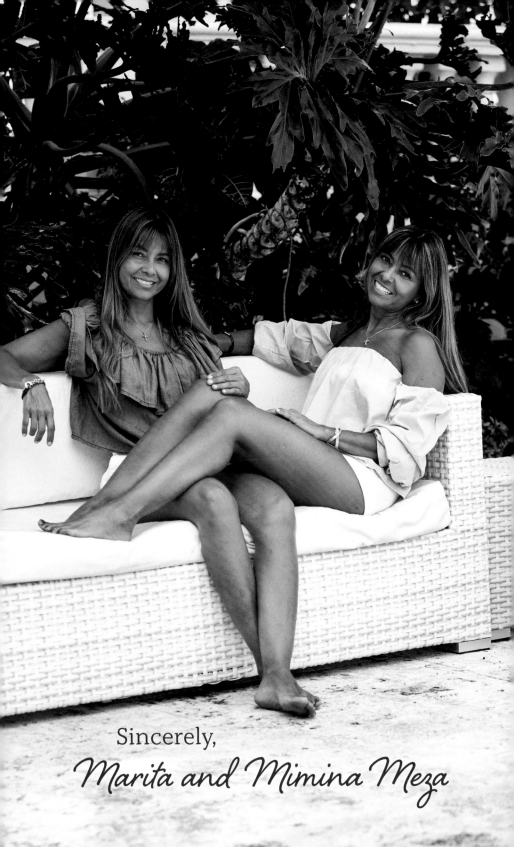

Sincerely,

Marita and Mimina Meza

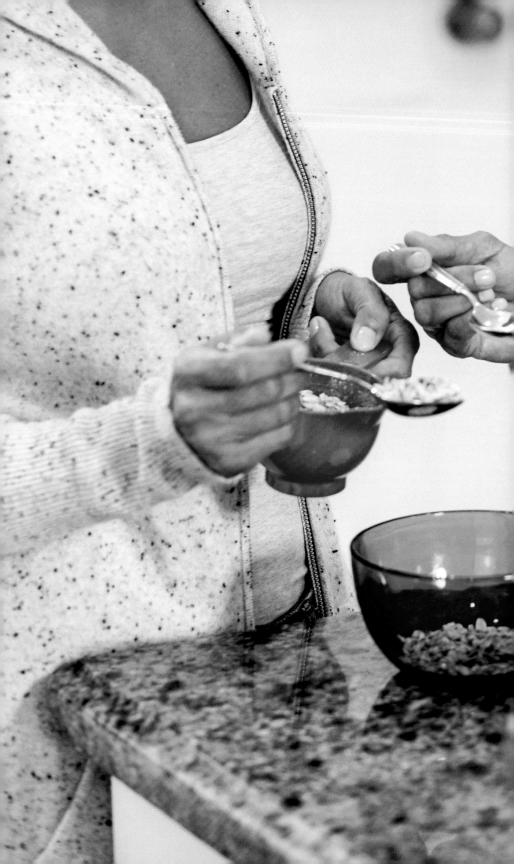

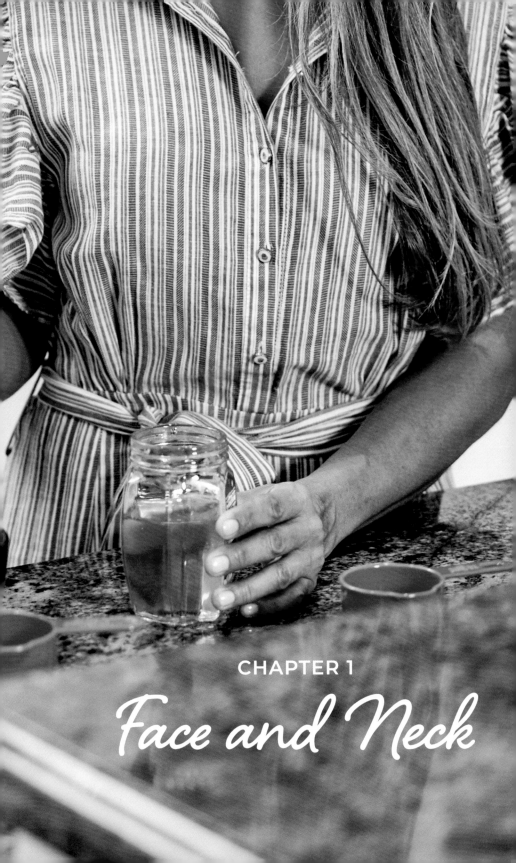

CHAPTER 1

Face and Neck

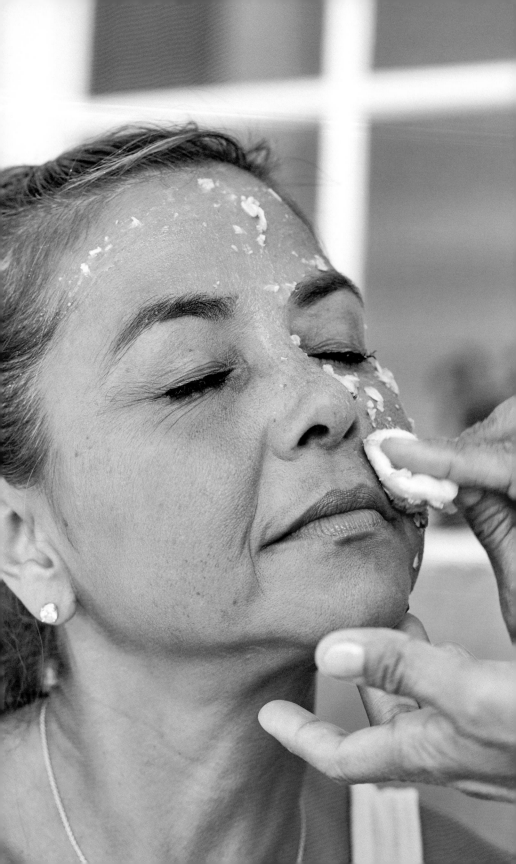

Face and Neck

Let's start with the most important parts of your body: your beautiful, fresh face and your gorgeous neck. In Spanish, we say, "La primera impression es la que vale," meaning the first impression is the most important. Your face is your first impression, so it's important to take extra good care of it.

But as you focus on taking care of your face, don't forget about your neck! It's so common for women to spend time and money cleansing, moisturizing, and protecting their face from the sun, while totally ignoring their neck. When you reach a certain age, all those years of taking care of skin in one area and ignoring another can become quite obvious, especially since the skin on your neck loses elasticity faster than skin on other parts of your body. Let's start thinking of the neck as an extension of the face. When you give your face some love, extend that love on down.

There are three important steps for a beautiful face and neck: cleaning, toning, and hydrating. We love using our secret recipes for homemade masks for all of these skin-care steps, and we are excited to share our recipes with you!

SALIVA

Before we get into the beauty recipes, we want to share an unusual trick using the power of your own saliva. Though it may sound gross, putting saliva on your face and neck really works to prevent wrinkles, acne, scars, spots, and even warts. Making sure your hands are clean first, lick your fingers and apply your saliva under and around your eyes and on the corners of your mouth. Leave it on for at least 20 minutes and then rinse off with a natural product and water.

A saliva-wash may sound like witchcraft, but it's instinctual to animals. They clean themselves with saliva and lick their wounds to heal themselves. Saliva acts like a curative agent. It has a chemical substance that helps to heal skin abrasions and irritations, and a protein that helps lower any chances of infection. If you're surprised by this remedy and hesitant to try it, trust us, it works. It's amazing that the substances we need are so readily available to us.

Most of our masks and treatments in this book can be made with ingredients you already have around your home. We've found that the recipes work for all types of skin, although you may find a particular recipe works especially well for you. Since most of our beauty treatments are made with fresh, perishable ingredients, we recommend making them each time you want to use them and throwing away any extra. When you can make a quantity and store it, we will specify that in the recipe.

CLEANSING

Cleansing your face seems pretty straightforward. After all, you've been doing it for years, probably with very little thought. But before you cleanse, if you wear makeup, you should use a natural makeup remover to remove *most* of your makeup, enabling your cleanser to do a better job. If you wear makeup on your neck, even extending your foundation past your jawline, don't forget to cleanse there as well. Your pores clog just as easily on your neck as on your face.

It's important to know that all cleansers are not created equal. They do not all work the same way at removing makeup and pollution to truly cleanse the skin. Depending on the ingredients, cleansers can cause irritation, dry skin, and even breakouts. So how do you properly wash your face? We recommend using a mild, natural soap made specifically for faces. Stay away from unnecessary foaming agents and artificial fragrances. It's a good idea to use facial cleanser on your neck as well, instead of body soap. The skin on the neck is similar to skin on the face, so it's best to use a gentle soap.

Water quality and temperature are also important for cleansing. When we were little girls, we grew up washing our faces in fresh, cold water from a mountain stream. It sounds very picturesque, but no, we didn't stick our faces directly into the stream every morning! Our house just happened to have access to fresh, crystalline, local water. We always found it refreshing to wash with cold water rather than hot. Now that we live in Miami, we continue using cold water, and we think it works better at keeping our skin hydrated.

In addition to cold water, ice can also help your face and neck look beautiful. Rubbing an ice cube on your skin for 15 seconds will help minimize open pores, making the skin look fresh and dewy. We try to do this every day. After all, it only takes 15 seconds!

Indulge yourself every day. Get a new hairstyle, eat your favorite ice cream, or go out of the way to spend time with friends and family. Do something to make yourself happy every single day.

HOW YOU WASH

The way you wash your face is almost as important as the products you use. It's easy to give your face a quick rub and be done with it, but a quick rub doesn't work to really cleanse your face. It's best to massage your face with cleanser for at least 30 seconds. Using your fingertips, rub in a gentle, circular motion to help dirt, oil, and buildup break free. Some women also find that a cleansing brush or cloth work better, but be aware that these tools perform exfoliation, which isn't needed every day. Exfoliating is a great way to cleanse skin even deeper, removing impurities that have settled deep into the skin, while sloughing off dead, dull skin cells. We recommend exfoliating your face and neck once or twice a week. It can reduce the appearance of wrinkles, improve your skin's texture, and clear up acne.

RICE WATER CLEANSE

- The extra water left in the pot after you cook rice

The next time you cook rice, add a little extra water to cleanse your face with. Rice water does wonders for your skin because it's enriched with vitamin B1. Rinsing your face with rice water makes your skin feel super soft and clean while helping you fight the aging process. For a porcelain complexion, try this monthly.

TONING

Many people aren't totally sure what toners are and why they're valuable. Toners are essentially how you complete the cleansing process. Since it's hard to fully remove impurities from your face with just a cleanser, toners have the extra muscle to leave your face totally clean.

Toners can vary a lot in terms of ingredients, but you should get one that works for your skin type. Some toners contain alcohol, which helps reduce oil and kill bacteria. Others hydrate, calm, and sooth the skin.

APPLE CIDER VINEGAR TONER

- 1 tablespoon apple cider vinegar
- 1 tablespoon filtered water

Mix and apply to the face and neck with a cotton round after cleansing. (This recipe is good for normal to oily skin, but you can adjust it to include a smaller ratio of vinegar if you have drier skin, such as a 1 to 4 ratio.) This Apple Cider Vinegar (ACV) toner protects your skin from premature aging, leaving your face and neck looking healthy and radiant. You can also try the recipe as spot-treatment for acne and dark marks.

This is the first of our many suggested uses for apple cider vinegar! In fact, we use it so much in this book, we're going to call it ACV from here forward. ACV does so many amazing things for your skin: fights acne, regulates the PH level in your skin, promotes better circulation, removes dead skin cells, regenerates skin tissue, and fully cleanses due to natural antibacterial properties. ACV is also known for having a subtle bleaching effect, improving the appearance of age/sun spots, acne scars, and pimples.

PORE-SHRINKING MASK

- ½ cup oats
- 2 egg whites

Mix and apply to your face and neck for about 20 minutes. Rinse off with warm water. A major benefit of egg whites is that they tighten and close up large pores. Eggs also have astringent properties that help to shrink pores by tightening the skin.

MOISTURIZING

It is essential to keep your skin hydrated. Moisturize your face and neck down to your chest every single morning with a moisturizer that is at least SPF 15. Keep in mind that sun damage can be worse where your skin is thinnest, and the neck and décolletage tend to have very sensitive skin. Religiously applying an SPF moisturizer is critical if you want to look 20 years younger and more beautiful!

Apply an intensive eye cream around your eyes and a rejuvenating cream over your face and neck.

MILK AND FLOWERS MASK

- 6 cups of milk
- 3 spoons of chamomile flower or elderflower

Mix the flower into the milk and let it soak for one hour. Warm the mixture gently on the stovetop without making it hot. Remove from heat and let cool. Strain the flowers from the milk and put the product in a bottle. Apply to your face for about 15 to 20 minutes, then rinse off with cold water.

Milk rejuvenates your skin, making it soft, and chamomile relaxes it.

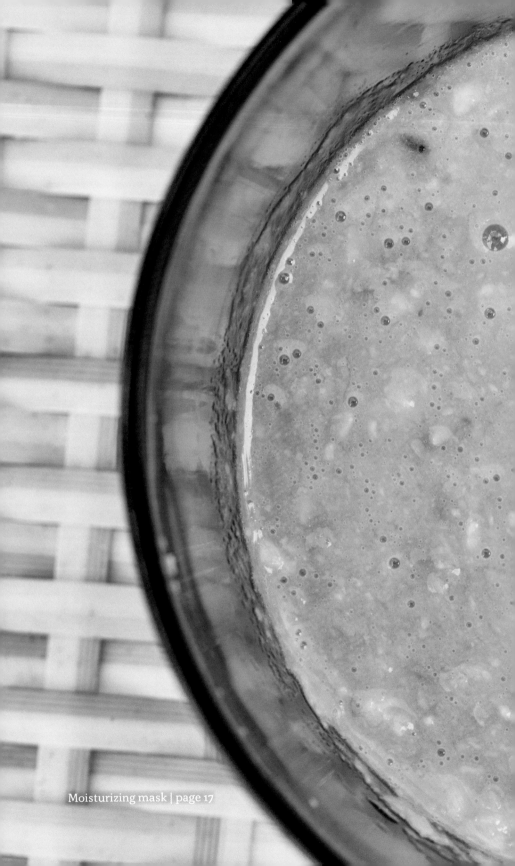

MOISTURIZING MASK

- A few drops of olive oil
- ½ cup of lemon juice
- 1 avocado

Mix all the ingredients. This is easiest with a blender or food processor, but it can be done by hand. Apply to your face for about 10 to 15 minutes, then rinse off with water.

This mask is perfect for women with dry skin and for staying moisturized in cold winter months.

THE MAGIC MASK

- ½ cup of oats
- 3 tablespoons of honey

Mix with a spoon and apply to your face and neck for about 20 minutes. Rinse off with warm water.

This secret recipe is our favorite! We were excited to discover this mask because it always makes our faces so soft and beautiful. Oats cleanse your skin and moisturize at the same time, while helping to regulate your pH. Because honey is naturally antibacterial, it's great for acne treatment and age prevention. This mask will make your face glow!

To be truly happy, you should focus on collecting experiences instead of material possessions. Experiences can be free. Spend an afternoon with someone you love or sit on a beach by yourself. Give value to moments rather than to things.

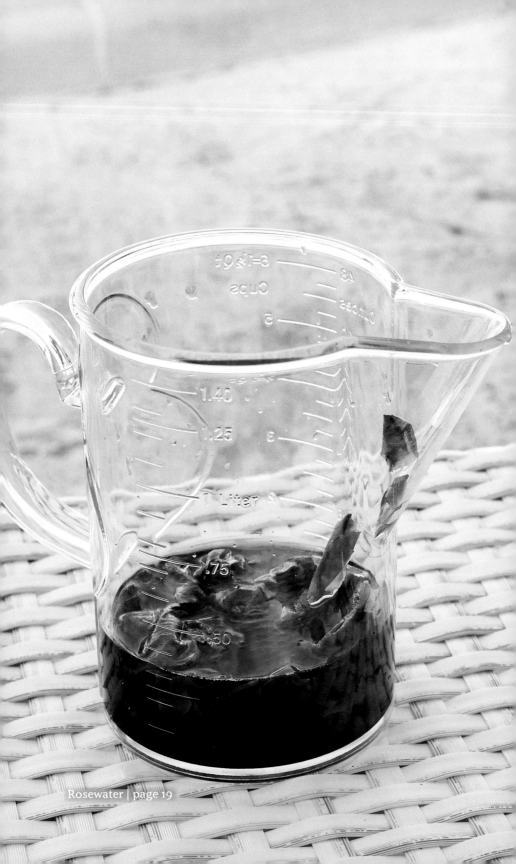

ROSEWATER

Women dream of soft, clean skin, and one of the secrets is rosewater. It's been around for generations, and the benefits are amazing! Roses help to firm the skin, accelerate healing, and decrease the appearance of stretch marks. The high content of vitamin C stimulates the production of collagen and protects the skin from free radicals, fighting the signs of aging. You can make rosewater with either dry or fresh rose petals.

 Dry Petals:
- 1/4 cup dry petals
- 1 1/4 cups distilled water

Using warm (not hot) water, add the dry petals and soak them for 10 to 15 minutes. When the water reaches room temperature, use a strainer to remove the petals, pouring the water of roses into a glass container. You can keep it for up to one week in the refrigerator.

 Fresh Petals:
- 1 cup of fresh rose petals (2 roses)
- 2 cups of distilled water
- 1 tablespoon of vodka

This recipe works best when roses are very fresh. Start by rinsing the petals. Add the water and vodka to a sauté pan on the stovetop. Evenly distribute the petals into the pan and simmer gently for 20 minutes without bringing to a full boil. Remove the mixture from the heat. When the water reaches room temperature, use a strainer to remove the petals, pouring the rosewater into a glass container. You'll see that the water has taken on the beautiful color of the roses. You can keep it for up to one week in the refrigerator.

 Uses:
- As a nightly rejuvenator, apply directly to the face and neck with a cotton ball before you go to sleep.

- Put the water in a little spray bottle and keep it in your refrigerator, misting your face whenever your skin needs a refresher.
- Reduce bags under the eyes by applying the rosewater to cotton rounds and leaving on the eye area for 10 minutes.
- Have a headache? Wet a washcloth with the rosewater and lie down with it on your forehead for 15 minutes. You'll feel your headache melt away.
- To relax at the end of the day, add a cup or two of rosewater to your bath. The fragrance has powerful stress-relieving properties.

ROSE MAKEUP REMOVER

- 2 tablespoons of warm coconut oil
- ½ cup rosewater

Mix ingredients together until smooth. Apply to your face in a gentle circular motion to remove even waterproof makeup. Wash your face with warm water and continue your nightly beauty routine.

ROSE FACE MASK

- 1 spoon of plain yogurt
- Rosewater

Mix and apply directly to your face for few minutes. Rinse off with cold water.

Water of roses opens your pores, and the fermentation in the yogurt is great for the skin.

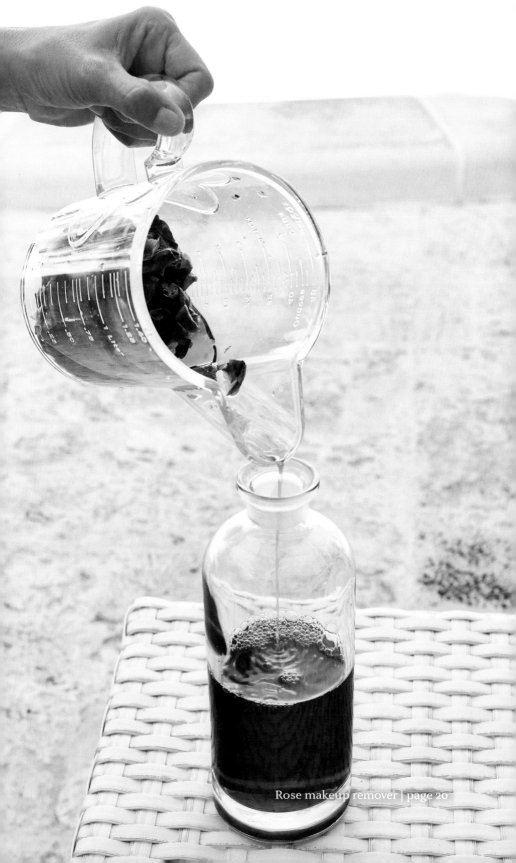

Rose makeup remover | page 20

THE SECRET WEAPON FOR PUFFY EYES

We have a surprising secret weapon for puffy eyes: hemorrhoid cream. Yes, we know it sounds crazy, but it really works for relieving swelling! (That's what's it's made for, albeit for a different part of your body!) It's best used the night before you need your eyes de-puffed. If you've been crying, not sleeping well, or tending toward puffiness for what-ever circumstances, apply a little hemorrhoid cream before you go to bed. It will also temporarily help reduce the appearance of wrinkles around the eye. This beauty secret works so well that you might want to keep doing it, but remember that it is not a substitute for regular night cream. It has powerful short-term ingredients, but you want treatments that help for the long term.

WRINKLE-FIGHTING CREAM

- 2 stems of aloe vera
- 1 egg white
- A couple leaves of fresh oregano

In a blender, mix the inside of the aloe vera with the rest of the ingre-dients until it's creamy. Apply to the whole neck for about 20 minutes and then wash off.

Aloe vera is a magical plant with wrinkle-fighting ingredients. Instead of paying a fortune for beauty creams that use aloe as the key ingredient, try this inexpensive homemade cream. You'll see how much you'll love it!

MASK FOR REDUCING LINES

- 1 egg white
- 1 teaspoon of honey

Mix ingredients and apply to the face and neck with a soft makeup brush. Leave for 10 to 12 minutes and wash off with lukewarm water. This mask will remove fine lines around your neck.

We use this one all the time! The honey makes you look like you just had a face lift. When you mix with the protein of the egg white, you look as if you've removed 2 to 3 years from your face.

PUMPKIN TREATMENT

- Organic canned pumpkin puree or fresh mashed pumpkin

Apply to the face and neck for 20 minutes, 3 or 4 times a week. Pumpkin is a great anti-aging vegetable. (We also include it in our diet!)

Don't hold grudges. Instead of carrying the weight of anger, forgive people who hurt you. This does not mean you need to let people who hurt you back into your life. But if you can release the negative feelings, you will live a happier life.

TIPS FOR A YOUNGER-LOOKING NECK

1. Stop looking down at your phone. It's doing more damage than you think: it leads to saggy jowls!

2. Sleep the right way. When you sleep on your back, you can minimize wrinkles on your face, neck, and chest because your skin isn't being squished and pulled during the night.

3. Do neck exercises. The neck has muscles that can be toned just like everywhere else on your body. When you tone these muscles, you can fight off sagginess and double chin. Yoga has many poses that work the neck and shoulders to keep your décolletage looking young and beautiful. You can also try our favorite exercise, which is a little hard to describe but easy to feel when it's working. Sit or stand up straight, open your mouth slightly, and tilt your head up a bit. Pull your lips tight against your teeth, almost like you're making a grimace. Engage the muscles in your neck, making a slow chewing motion. You should feel the tension in your muscles and tendons. We do this exercise for a few minutes every morning while we're getting ready.

4. Neck massages feel great, but make sure you don't over-massage the skin on the neck. It is very thin and super delicate—even more delicate than the skin on your face. When you or someone else massages your neck, it can stretch the skin, ultimately making it lose elasticity. You can still massage your neck, but make sure you do it gently. The proper way to massage the neck is by moving

both your palms from lower to upper region in vertical movements. Never massage your neck in circular motions or from top to bottom. Keep this advice in mind when you apply lotion, exfoliate, or wash your neck.

5. If you use other types of masks, avoid letting them dry and crack on your neck. Fruit-based masks are okay, but masks that contain ingredients like clay, flour, and mud can dry and be hard to remove from your delicate skin.

Don't compare yourself with others. The beauty in this world is that we are all different from each other. So what if your friend is richer than you? Riches don't mean anything. As our father always said, "Happiness isn't about who is richer, but who needs less." When you live without envy, you are rich in this world.

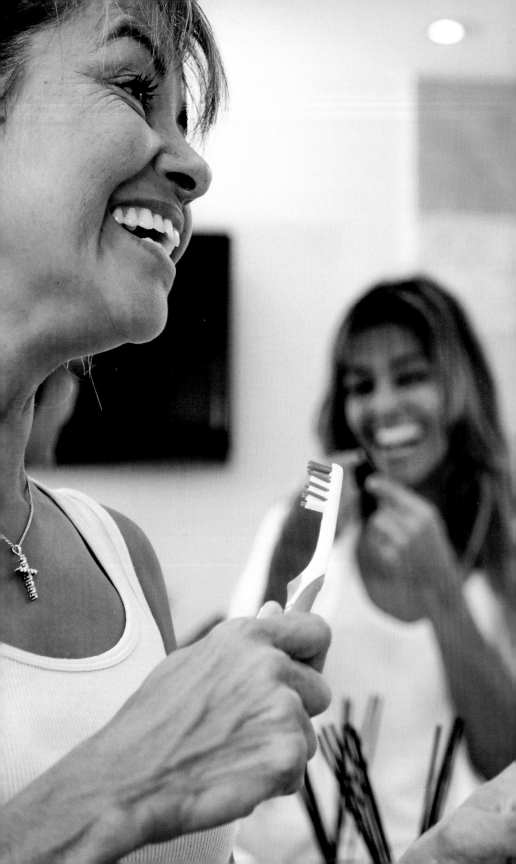

CHAPTER 2

Smile

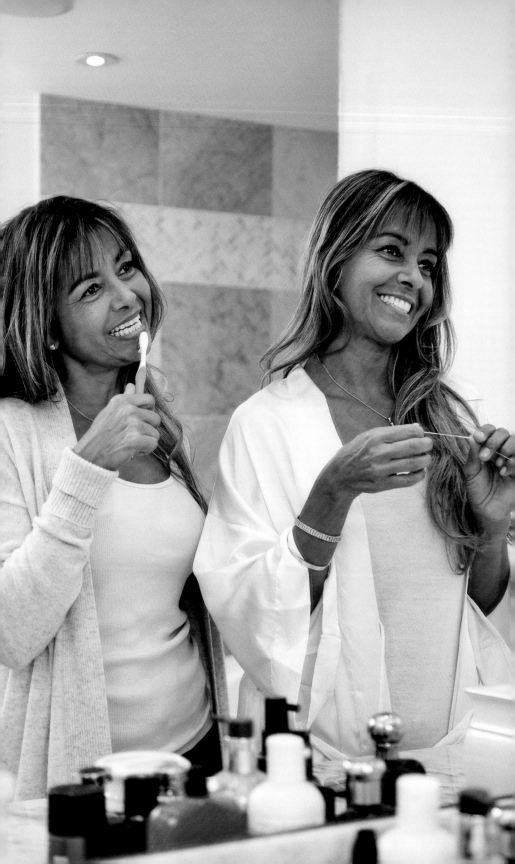

Smile

People always ask how we keep our teeth so white. It's hard because so many delicious foods and drinks can stain them! Our first beauty secret isn't really a secret: we try to brush our teeth and gums after every meal or snack. We don't like food or drinks to sit on our teeth because it can cause staining and cavities.

We recommend a toothpaste that contains baking soda and enhanced plaque removal. We find this kind of toothpaste works significantly better than non-baking soda toothpaste. In the evening, we also floss before we brush and use mouthwash after to freshen our breath and prevent plaque.

Aside from that, we have a few secrets to share to help you keep your teeth super white and clean!

EXTRA SPARKLE TOOTHPASTE

- A pinch of baking soda
- A few drops of lemon juice

Mix into a paste and scoop some onto your toothbrush. Before you go to bed, give your teeth a good brush. Do this once a month, and you'll see the difference! Baking soda is a mild abrasive, and it gently scrubs away stains leaving your smile sparkly white.

BREATH-FRESHENING MOUTHWASH

- 1/2 teaspoon of baking soda
- 1 glass of water

Mix together and use like mouthwash. Baking soda can help rebalance the level of acid in your mouth, preventing bad breath.

TREATMENT FOR BLEEDING GUMS

- Aloe vera
- Mint
- 1 spoonful of baking soda

Mix all of the ingredients and brush your teeth to reduce harmful bacteria and inflammation of the gums.

A Note on Baking Soda: Baking soda really is a miracle product, but you have to be careful! It's an alkaline substance, so when it mixes with an acid, it alters pH levels. Over-exposure to alkaline substances can burn your skin, or in this case, irritate your mouth. It can also damage enamel and increase temperature sensitivity if overused. So, no matter how much you love our baking soda recipes, don't use them every day! Experts recommend using baking soda for your teeth no more than twice a week.

Stress is bad for both physical and mental health. Focus on the things you can change instead of wasting energy worrying about the things that are out of your control.

TIPS FOR BEAUTIFUL TEETH

- Don't brush your teeth right after you drink coffee. The acid in coffee can soften enamel that can brush away in small amounts, which can turn into significant amounts over time. It's also believed that using toothpaste right after drinking coffee can make stains sink in more. After drinking coffee, it's best to rinse your mouth with water and wait at least 30 minutes before you brush.
- Limit the amount of dark liquids you drink, such as coffee, tea, and soda. When you do drink liquids that are more likely to stain your teeth, use a straw. This helps the liquid bypass your front teeth so that they stay whiter. You can buy metal straws to use at home for hot beverages.
- Limit the amount of sugar in your diet. A diet high in sugar supports the growth of bacteria, which causes plaque and gingivitis.
- Don't smoke! Aside from the many other health concerns, smoking makes your teeth yellow.
- Get a new toothbrush. Electric toothbrushes are a great option for ensuring a deep scrub, but make sure you get one with a round, oscillating head.
- Eat crunchy foods that naturally clean the teeth as you chew, such as apples, raw veggies, nuts, and seeds. When you know you can't brush right after eating, these are great foods to finish your meal with.

- Go to the dentist every 6 months. Getting your teeth cleaned professionally on a regular basis will help you prevent cavities and ensure a whiter smile!

We started modeling at 12 years old, and our teeth were perfectly white! The challenge has been keeping our smiles beautiful over the years. The recipes and tips in this chapter have really helped us, and we hope they will help you too!

Cultivate your inner beauty. When you are beautiful inside, it is a reflection of your soul and people notice immediately. Even strangers can see your virtues: your enthusiasm, your sense of humor, and your interest to help others. They can also see the love you radiate to your family, work, pets, and self. To project a truly positive image, beauty must come from the inside.

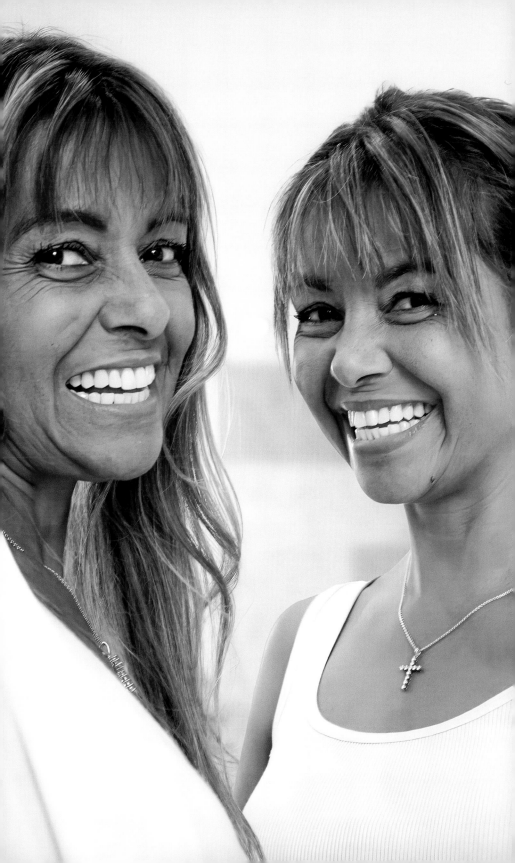

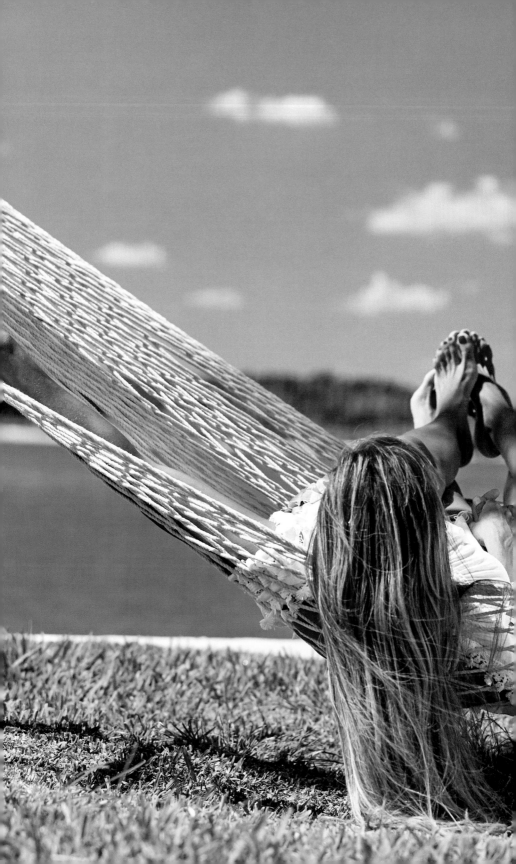

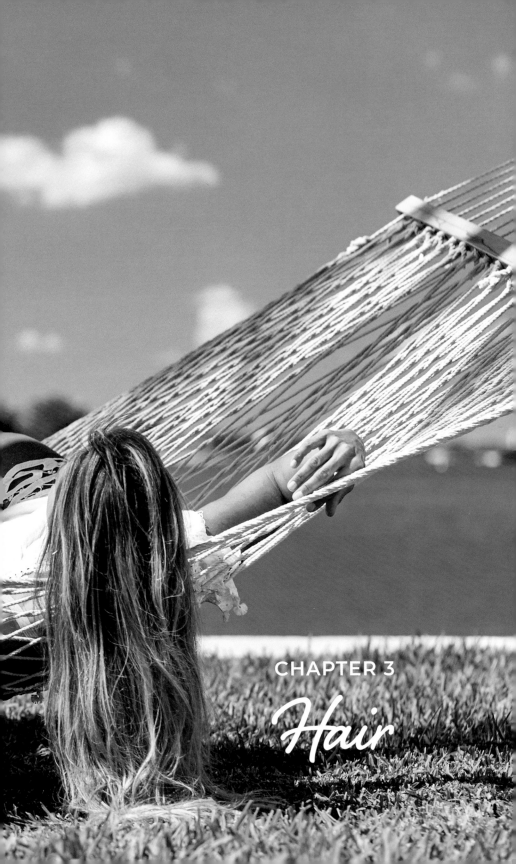

CHAPTER 3

Hair

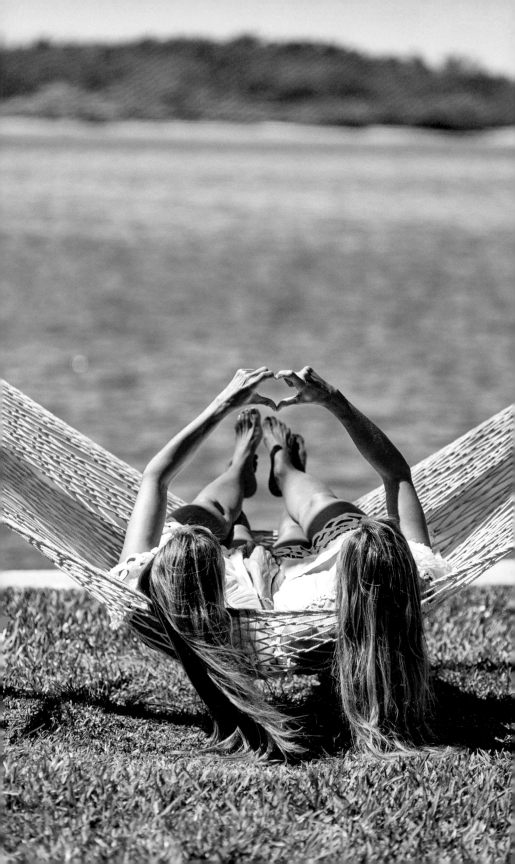

Hair

A lot of people think we're either born with naturally healthy, beautiful hair or destined to have unhealthy hair. This is not true! Just like the rest of our bodies, we must take care of our hair. Over the years, we have noticed that our hair looks much better when we keep it healthy. It grows longer faster, it's shinier, it has more volume, and it's easier to style. When we don't put in the effort, it's easy to see the difference.

As a woman, you know that when your hair looks amazing, everything else seems to fall into place! That's why taking care of your hair is one of the easiest ways to look your best. Here are our best secrets for beautiful, ageless hair.

Nutrition: Healthy hair starts with a healthy body. Eating nutritious foods and drinking plenty of water is essential for healthy hair. Vitamins are also important, and we recommend taking a multivitamin every day. Taking biotin as a supplement is also very effective for growing hair faster.

WASHING

Washing your hair seems so basic. You've been doing it your whole life; surely you must be doing it right! But chances are, you could change a few things to wash your hair better.

Let's start with how often to wash. Hair is a lot like skin: it is important to know your level of dryness/oiliness so that you can treat it appropriately. Most women don't need to wash their hair every day. You might find that by washing your hair slightly less often, it looks healthier. It seems counterintuitive, but this is even true for women who have oily hair. When you wash oily hair every day, your body can respond by producing more oil to make up for the amount that's lost during washing. When they switch to washing every other day, many women find that their scalp stops producing so much oil, and their hair looks healthier. Just note that it may take a few weeks for the scalp to adjust.

In addition, make sure you find the right shampoo. Choose products for your particular hair type, whether it's curly, fine, color-treated, or damaged. We have curly hair, and we find that shampoo for curls really does make a difference.

When it comes to applying shampoo, you might be surprised that you could be doing it wrong. A lot of women have such thick hair that they don't properly wash their scalp, causing serious product build-up, especially if you use hard-to-remove products such as dry shampoo. When you wash your hair, remember that you need to thoroughly wash your scalp too. To massage shampoo over your entire scalp, you may need to add water as you wash. Clean roots are healthy for your hair, and healthy hair grows faster and looks better.

After washing, don't forget the conditioner! Most women should be using conditioner on the ends of their hair every time they wash it. Avoid rubbing conditioner into your scalp—it combines with your natural scalp oils to make your hair look greasy and weighed down.

Water temperature is also important. We love to take hot showers, but hot water can strip the scalp of essential oils, making hair feel drier and look duller. And as with oily hair, drying out the scalp can actually increase oil production. When we want to take a super-hot shower, we stand under the showerhead with our body but wait to wash our hair until we turn the temperature down a bit.

Rinsing with cold water helps seal the hair cuticle, making it lay more smoothly. Smooth hair reflects light better so that it looks shinier.

Don't be so hard on yourself when you make a mistake. Everyone makes mistakes. Humans are perfectly imperfect, and that's what makes life beautiful. Mistakes are a way to learn, grow, and ultimately boost your confidence.

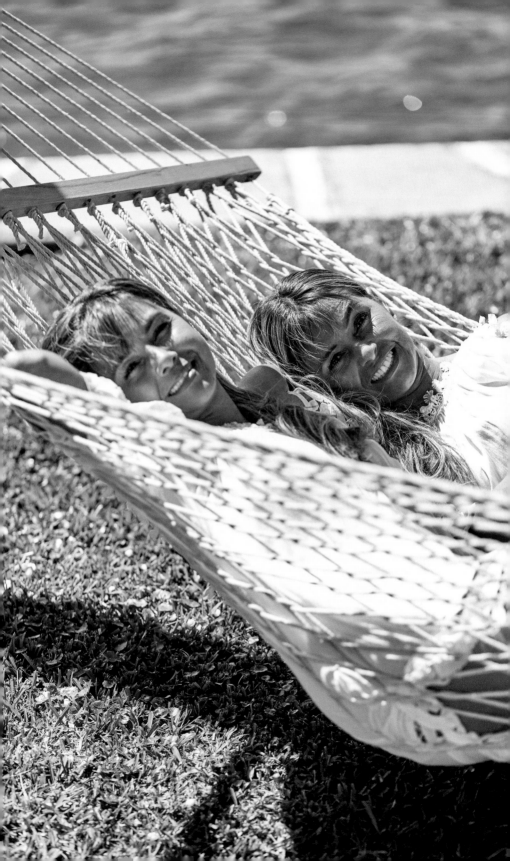

BRUSHING

There are many different kinds of hairbrushes, and it's important to use the appropriate type for your hair. For example, a boar-bristle brush helps distribute natural oils from your scalp through the rest of your hair, so it's great for women with dry hair but bad for women with oily hair. Most importantly, you want a brush that will gently remove tangles without pulling too hard on the roots or breaking it off mid-strand. We use a wet brush. It runs effortlessly through our hair, detangling without pulling or tugging. You can use it on wet or dry hair, and it's great for all types—curly or straight, thick or fine.

TREATMENTS

Most women spend time washing and styling their hair, but they don't spend much time on treatments. At-home treatments can actually make a huge difference in how your hair looks and feels! We love that these recipes are inexpensive and easy to do without going to a salon. We strongly believe in natural hair treatment because a lot of products out there have many chemicals that can damage your hair and health. We love the recipes in this chapter and hope you do too!

MASK FOR SPLIT ENDS

- 2 tablespoons of olive oil
- 1 tablespoon of honey
- 1 egg

Mix and apply only to the ends of your hair. Leave on for about 30 minutes, then remove with warm water. This formula works for all types of hair and can be used once every two weeks.

It's hard to find all-natural products that make your hair look healthy and shiny, but this one works! Olive oil helps moisturize split ends. When it combines with the honey and egg, it adds softness and shine.

A Note on Lemons: Lemons are a natural miracle product for your hair and scalp! Because they are acidic, they can effectively cleanse the scalp of dead cells. They also have anti-fungal properties that fight dandruff and other scalp infections, and they're a rich source of Vitamin C, which helps make hair long and strong. That said, lemons should be used in moderation. Because they are acidic, excessive use can make hair dry and brittle. Also remember that lemon alone is a bleaching agent. Unless you are trying to make your hair color lighter, do not leave pure lemon juice on your hair for more than 10 minutes.

HAIR GROWTH MASK

- A few drops of essential lemon oil (not lemon juice)
- 1 teaspoon castor oil
- 1 teaspoon warm olive oil

Mix and massage well into your scalp and hair for 5 to 10 minutes. Leave overnight. In the morning, continue with the lemon juice hair therapy and wash using an herbal shampoo.

Castor oil helps grow hair, and the other oils add supporting nutrients.

HAIR GROWTH VINEGAR TREATMENT

- 1 cup ACV
- 2 cups filtered water

Pour ingredients into a spray bottle. Wash and condition your hair as you normally would, then spray the mixture onto your hair and wait 10 minutes before rinsing. ACV will make your hair grow like crazy. It regulates the PH value of your scalp, preventing dandruff, relieving itchiness, and removing dead skin cells that clog hair follicles. ACV also helps naturally remove product buildup in your hair. If your hair is dry or dyed, this might not be the best treatment for you, as it can have a drying effect.

LEMON AND ALOE VERA MOISTURE MASK

- 2 tablespoons of fresh, natural aloe vera gel. (If you have an aloe plant, you can cut off a chunk and scoop out the aloe.)
- 1 tablespoon of fresh lemon juice

Mix well and spend 5 minutes massaging it into your scalp and hair. Wait for 20 to 30 minutes and rise off with water. You can shampoo and condition your hair as you usually would.

DEEP CONDITIONER FOR DAMAGED HAIR

- ½ banana (or plantain)
- 1 avocado
- 1 egg
- 2 tablespoons of extra virgin olive oil

Mix the banana, olive oil, and avocado until the ingredients are well incorporated. Next, add the egg and mix until you have a soft texture. Apply to damp hair, without touching the scalp. Wait for 10 to 15 minutes and wash off with warm water only.

This recipe is amazing because all of the ingredients play an important role in improving your hair's health. Bananas and plantains fight frizz, while avocado helps to hydrate hair and promote its growth. Olive oil makes hair strong and shiny, and egg makes hair shiny and soft. With all of these ingredients combined, you can't find a better deep conditioner!

The people you let into your life should make you feel good about yourself. Do a gut-check on your circle of friends and loved ones. If they make you feel worse about yourself or trigger that negative voice in your head, maybe it's time to end those relationships so you can surround yourself with positive, supportive people.

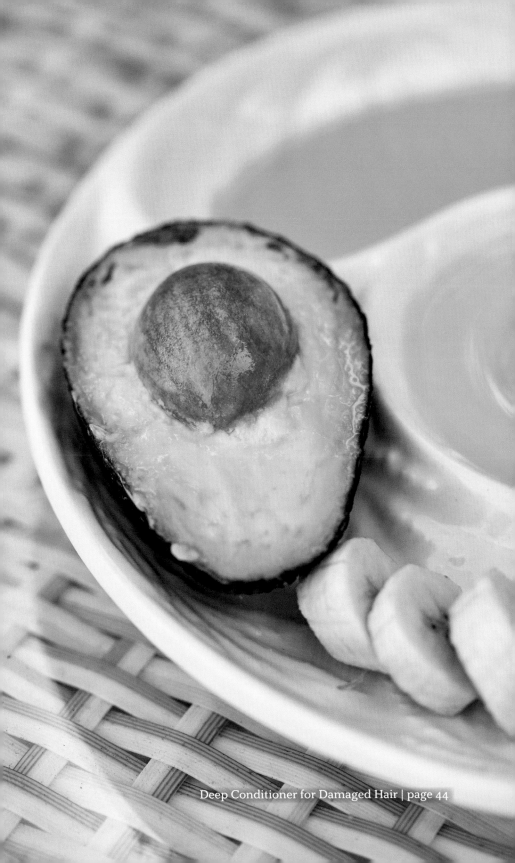

Deep Conditioner for Damaged Hair | page 44

AVOIDING BREAKAGE

Breakage is the enemy of beautiful hair. It creates frizz and fly-aways and makes it harder for your hair to grow. Luckily, there are many ways to be nicer to your hair!

- Sleep on a silk pillowcase, which creates a slippery surface for your hair, allowing it to move around instead of getting as tangled and roughed-up as it would on a cotton pillowcase. Silk helps prevent breakage and makes your hair easier to style in the morning.
- Get a quick-drying towel that's made specifically for hair. Typical towels aren't that absorbent, and you end up rubbing your hair more than you should. Short on cash? An old cotton T-shirt dries hair better than a typical towel.
- Wearing a ponytail every day can be hard on your hair, since hair ties can put extra stress on hair and cause breakage. Try wearing your hair down more often, getting soft hair ties, or positioning looser, lower ponytails.
- Be patient with tangles. Ripping at them is a surefire way to break your strands.

TIPS FOR BEAUTIFUL HAIR

- Avoid stress! A lot of women who go through traumatic and/ or high-stress periods in their lives notice significant hair thinning a few months after the incident. Luckily, hair typically grows back to its normal fullness as long as the stress subsides, but it's one more reason to stay calm.
- If your hair is thinning, be extra gentle with it. Avoid brushing it too roughly or when it's wet.
- The sun can damage hair. If you spend a lot of time outside, invest in some cute hats to protect your hair.
- To get more volume, part your hair on the opposite side of your head.
- Get your hair trimmed at least every three months to remove split ends and promote growth. If your hair grows slowly, get a micro-trim that cuts off only the split ends. If you have bangs, get them trimmed every few weeks. (As identical twins, we always went to the salon together so that our hair could be cut exactly the same!)
- Letting your hair dry naturally is best. When you need to use a blow-dryer, make sure it isn't too hot, especially close to your scalp.
- Massage your head for about 10 minutes every day or at least twice a week. Massaging releases your scalp's natural oils. (It also feels great! Have a friend or partner help.)

- Be aware of when your hair goes through situations that can cause extra stress and damage, like a day at the beach or big-city pollution. Give your hair extra love and bring it back to a beautiful state by doing some of these natural treatments.
- After washing your hair, apply a hair serum or weightless oil such as almond, coconut, or Moroccan oil. We like to apply a drop or two when our hair is wet to make it shinier and fuller.
- If you really want to promote hair growth, try a product called Natrol. We tried a ton of products before finding this one, and it really works! It also helps promote nail growth.

If you haven't been doing much to take care of your hair, all of these tips might seem like a lot to do, but they're all small changes that don't take much time. Try a few and see how they work for you. As you see the results, we bet you'll be inspired to keep going!

As identical twins, we've always looked alike, but we can both tell when one of us hasn't been taking care of her hair! We can style it the exact same way, but one of us will look better than the other! Having a busy lifestyle can make it hard to keep up with beauty routines, but having healthy hair that cooperates during styling can actually save you a lot of time and effort down the road!

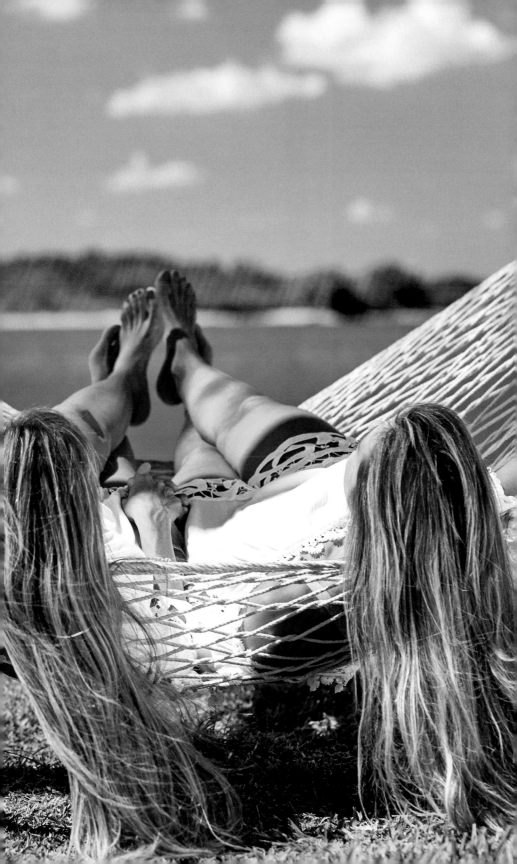

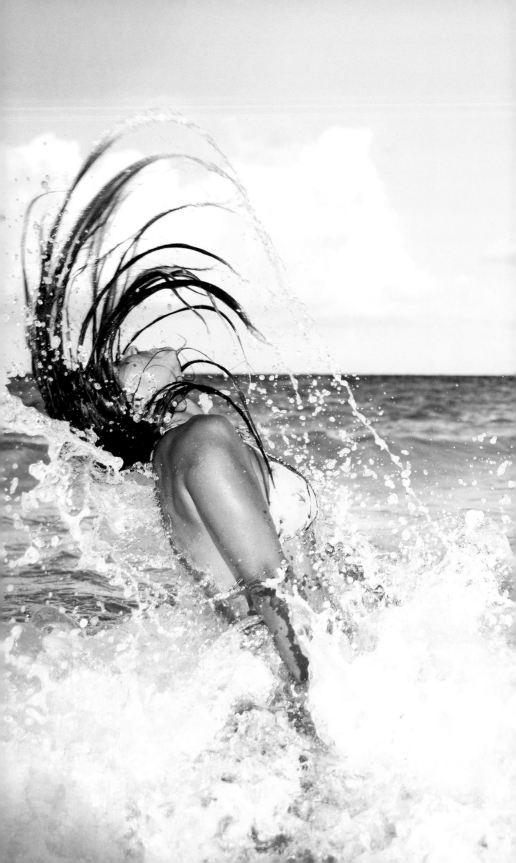

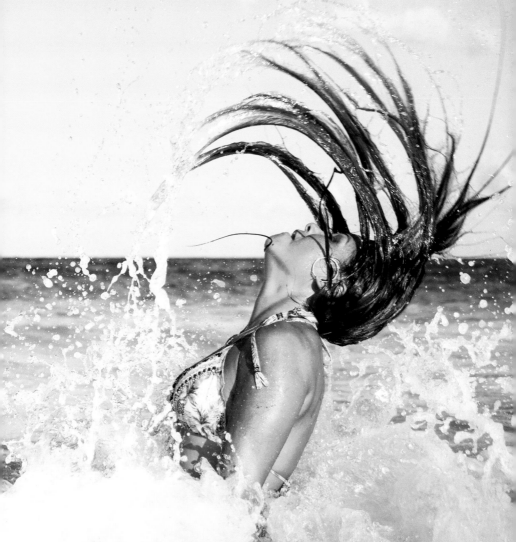

CHAPTER 4

Skin

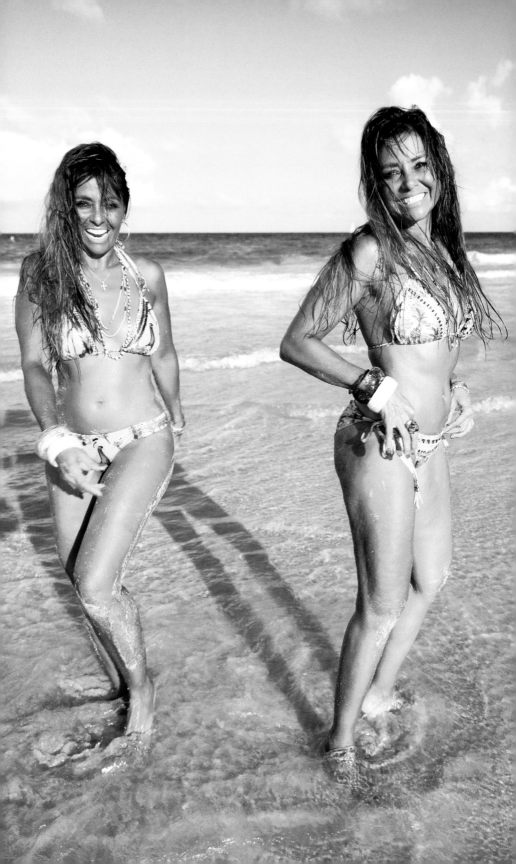

Skin

When it comes to looking younger and more beautiful, one of the most important things you can do is to take care of your skin. We talked about skincare a lot in "The Face and Neck" chapter, but that's just a small portion of your body's skin. As the largest organ of the body, the skin is the reflection of your overall health. It shows how much you drink or party, how much sleep you get, and how well you nourish yourself. When you take care of your overall health, your skin will show it.

That said, even when you take great care of your body, you probably have some problem areas with your skin. One of the most common (and dreaded) skin annoyances is cellulite. We hate to see those dimples across our beautiful skin! But no matter how much you work out, sometimes they just don't want to disappear from certain areas. Luckily, there are a few tricks for reducing their appearance, and they actually work!

The easiest thing you can do is to dry brush your skin. Dry brushing helps to eliminate excess liquid and toxins in your body by stimulating the lymphatic system, getting the blood flowing, and ultimately helping your skin look soft and smooth rather than dimpled. Get a brush with soft bristles and brush problem areas in a gentle, circular motion. It's best to do it for about five minutes twice a week before you shower. It's simple and really works! You can also exfoliate your skin with a variety of products. Caffeine is powerful ingredient to fight cellulite, so check out the at-home treatment below.

CELLULITE SCRUB

· **Coffee grounds**

When you brew your coffee, keep the grounds to use as a scrub for cellulite. We like to keep a little jar in our shower just for this purpose. You can rub a small amount on your legs, butt, stomach, or anywhere else that's showing signs of dimples. Just be careful of getting the coffee grounds down your shower drain. You can wipe the scrub off with a wet paper towel and throw it away after your shower to avoid getting the grounds down the drain. Rinse your body off with warm water and natural soap. It won't totally get rid of cellulite, but it helps. Trust us! Make sure you do it 3 or 4 times a week to see results.

CELLULITE-FIGHTING WATER

· **Edible calendula oil (you can find this in a natural products store)**

Mix 10 drops of edible calendula oil into a glass of water and drink.

You have to make a commitment with this one to see results, so we recommend drinking the Cellulite-Fighting Water every couple of days on an ongoing basis. Note that calendula is safe to consume, but it can irritate some gallbladder conditions, so consult your doctor before using it. This treatment is not for women who are pregnant or breastfeeding.

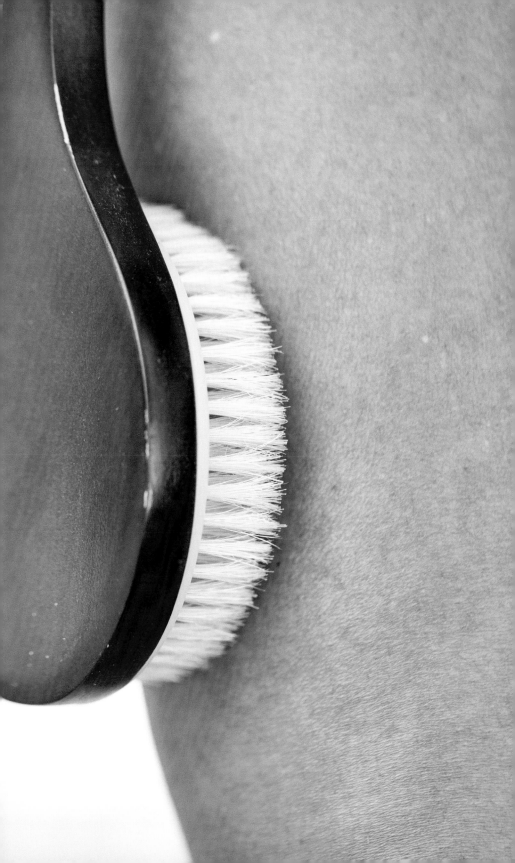

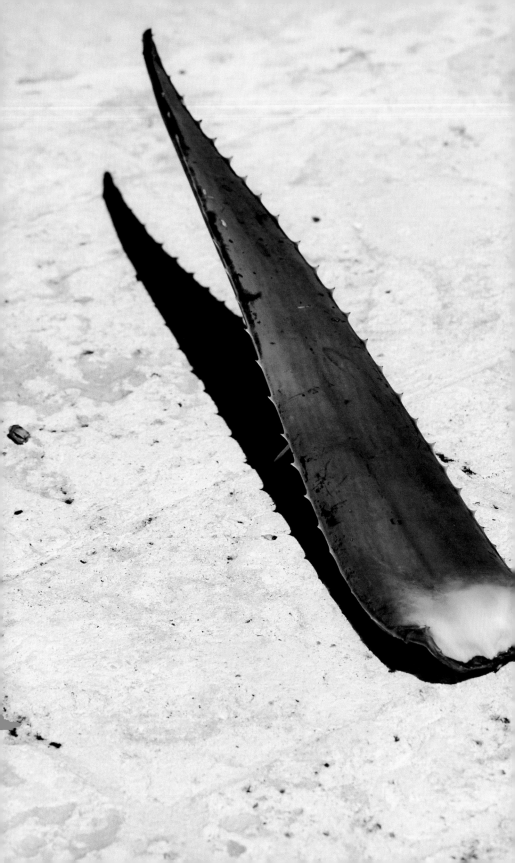

THE MANY WAYS TO USE ALOE VERA

- Wrinkles: Remove the skin of the aloe vera, then cut it in small pieces. Take two of those pieces and squeeze the juice to apply to your face and neck. Leave overnight. Massaging with aloe vera also has a rejuvenating effect.

- Wounds: Remove the skin of the plant and put it directly on the skin. Wrap the wound and leave it. The aloe stimulates cell regeneration and has antibacterial effects.

- Razor burn: Place the aloe vera under your arm after you shave and leave it overnight. The aloe vera's high moisture content is infused with anti-inflammatory properties.

- Dark Circles: Use a cotton round to apply aloe vera gel on dark patches in the morning to get a beautiful natural glow.

- Natural gloss: With a little brush, mix the gel of the aloe vera with your favorite liquid color and put it on your lips for a natural lip gloss.

- Messy hair: Use the gel directly on the area where your hair needs it.

- Oily skin: With a brush, mix aloe vera gel with your favorite foundation and apply to your face for a matte finish.

- Messy eyebrows: Use a clean eyelash brush and apply aloe gel on your eyebrows.

Feeling blue? Get moving! Exercise is proven to help improve your mood.

SECRETS TO KEEP YOUR SKIN HEALTHY AND BEAUTIFUL

1. Your skin is a 5.5 on the pH scale, but a lot of body products are much higher on the pH scale. Soaps that don't match your pH level can dry out your skin. You can even get eczema, rashes, and a whole range of issues on your lady parts, including yeast infections, bacterial infections, and general itchiness. Do a quick online search to check your soap's pH level and see if you need to buy something different.

2. Use products that contain the ingredients humectant and collagen.

3. Showers can actually dry out your skin, so use a good body cream after every shower to keep your skin hydrated and soft.

4. Wear sunscreen every day, even if you "don't burn." Don't sit in the sun between 11:30 a.m. and 2:30 p.m., when the rays are the strongest.

5. Use a homemade mask all over your body twice a month to avoid dry skin.

6. If you get a cut or wound, remember that the skin is usually very good at healing itself, but it must be hydrated to do so quickly. Drink extra water!

As you age, your skin is likely to change your total appearance more than anything else. Protecting and nourishing your skin will make a big difference in your appearance and expression lines, otherwise known as wrinkles. This is true for your face, neck, hands, arms, and every other part of your body!

Stretchmarks are another issue many women struggle with, particularly if they've experienced weight fluctuation or childbirth. Keeping the skin hydrated with good creams or oils will help it stretch in and out without causing scarring. But you have to be careful to select the right kind of oil. Choose oils that are light and pure. Olive oil, sweet almond oil, chamomile oil, eucalyptus oil, and rose oil are good options.

In addition to fighting stretchmarks and cellulite topically, you can fight them through your diet. Your body makes collagen naturally, which helps skin look young and beautiful. But by the time you reach your mid-twenties, your collagen production starts to decline. Luckily, there are foods you can eat that contain collagen and that increase your body's ability to produce it. For beautiful, younger-looking skin, add these foods to your diet: bone broth (e.g., ramen), eggs, salmon, kiwi, jelly, berries, avocado, cabbage, fish, beans, and garlic. These foods are especially important if you are pregnant or in the midst of dramatic weight fluctuation.

> You can't stop getting older, but you can continue looking younger and more beautiful if you take great care of your skin. The sooner you start, the better shape you'll be in later in life.

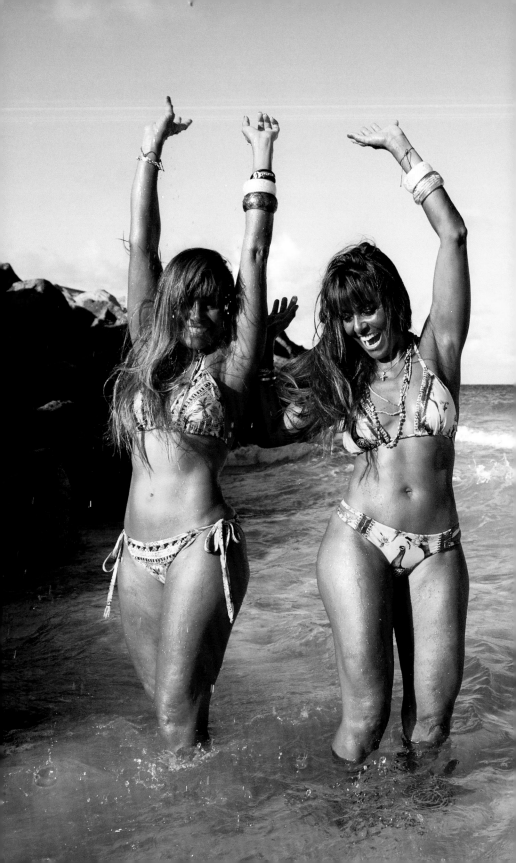

CHAPTER 5

Body

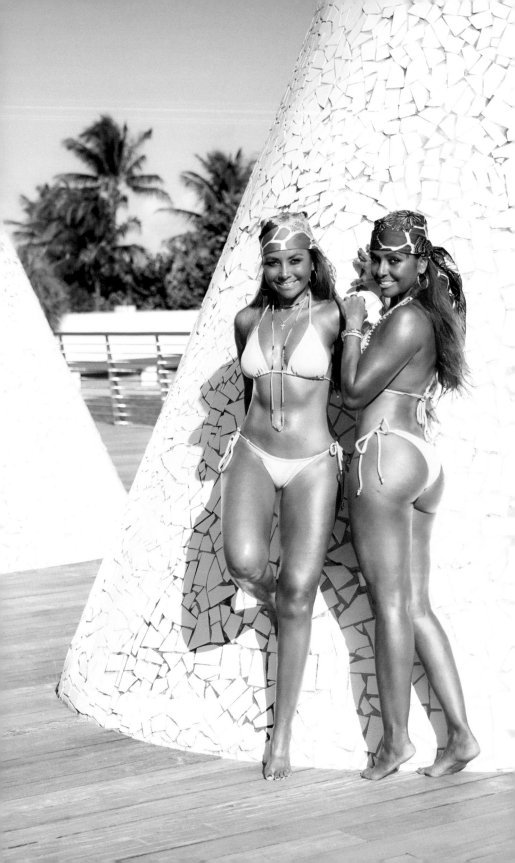

Body

When we wake up in the morning, we thank the Lord for one more day of life. Even if our bodies aren't perfect in our eyes, we are grateful to be alive and healthy.

We find that by focusing on health and gratitude, everything else seems to follow—especially beauty. Of course, we all want a beautiful body, but a beautiful body is one that functions as well as it possibly can. Our bodies allow us to do the things we love, like spending time with our friends, hiking, enjoying nature, and pursuing careers we find fulfilling.

Many times, people don't realize how important their health is until it's compromised. When you're sick or injured, it's easy to see how much more important health is than beauty. That's why this chapter is about overall wellness and how to stay healthy.

We all love to dream about what's possible in life, but it's much nicer when those dreams become true! When you put in the effort and have a positive attitude, you'll be amazed what you can achieve!

WATER

Let's talk about water! We drink water all day long, and we believe it's a key reason we stay healthy. Water is essential, and most people don't drink enough of it. Water might seem like a boring choice since it isn't the tastiest beverage, but it is the best for your body, skin, hair, and every other part of you! Sodas and sweet drinks contain water, but they are loaded with sugar and don't hydrate your body in the same way.

Water has an incredible number of benefits for your body:

1. Relieves fatigue. Fatigue is the first sign of dehydration, so if you feel tired, there's a good chance drinking more water would give you more energy.

2. Helps with headaches and migraines. When you get a headache, the first thing you should do is drink a big glass of water. It's amazing how often water alone is enough to make you feel better.

3. Aids digestion and constipation. If your body does not have enough of water, the colon pulls water from the stools in order to maintain hydration.

4. Encourages weight loss. Sometimes when you think you're hungry, you're really mistaking hunger for thirst. Drinking water can help keep you from overeating. Try to drink two glasses of water within a half hour before a meal to help curb your appetite.

5. Promotes healthy skin. Everyone desires glowing, dewy skin. You can get a smooth, youthful complexion by increasing your intake of H2O.

6. Eases a hangover. We know there is no quick fix to a long night of drinking alcohol, but consuming lots of water when you drink alcohol is a great way to lessen a hangover.

7. Fights bad breath. A dry mouth and a bad taste in your mouth can be signs of dehydration.

8. We find it extremely important to drink more than eight glasses of water daily (half a gallon), and we hope you do too! It is a must-do with no excuses—or as we call it in Spanish, *querer es poder*, meaning *wanting is power.*

BANANA TEA

- 2 bananas
- 1 liter of water

Bring the water to a boil. Wash the bananas, then cut both the fruit and skin into small pieces. Place in boiling water for 10 minutes. Strain and drink as a tea one hour before bedtime.

Bananas are rich in potassium and magnesium, but what a lot of people don't know is that the skin has even more potassium and magnesium than the fruit itself! Banana tea is great for soothing muscle aches and cramps and promoting heart health.

Our bodies are our temples, and we take care of them like our greatest treasure. There are a variety of ways we make our bodies a priority. The combination of water, good food, exercise, and sleep is especially important for staying healthy and looking young and beautiful.

NUTRITION AND VITAMINS

In addition to getting enough water, proper nutrition is a key factor in staying healthy. Eating an extremely balanced diet should provide most of the vitamins and minerals you need to keep your skin, hair, teeth, and nails beautiful.

We eat a lot of high-nutrient vegetables like broccoli, carrots, sweet potatoes, and leafy greens. We also eat high-nutrient fruits, like grapefruit, berries, avocado, and pineapple. Even though we want to stay slim, we don't shy away from eating fats, but we are picky about the kinds of fats we eat. Healthy fats like olive oil, nuts, and salmon are good for the body and keep us full so we don't snack in between meals. Bad fats like deep-fried foods are loaded with cholesterol and bad for the body.

There are many specific diets and weight-loss eating plans out there, and we encourage you to find whatever works for you. We believe the key is eating a wide variety of fruits and veggies, eating so that you feel satisfied, and not skipping meals. You want a diet you can maintain as a lifestyle, not something that takes all your energy and discipline for a few weeks and makes you rebound into an eating free-for-all.

Whatever healthy diet you choose, know that most people don't get the full amount of recommended vitamins and minerals. That's a problem, since vitamins not only keep us beautiful, but also help to safeguard us against illness and disease. That's why we swear by taking a good multivitamin. There is some controversy in whether multivitamins actually make a difference in a person's day-to-day wellness, but many studies have shown that various vitamins can fight specific health issues. We think of vitamins like an insurance policy. We try to eat the best we can to get our vitamins and minerals from food, and we also take a multivitamin just in case.

Get your multivitamin from a trusted supplier, since the vitamin industry isn't well regulated. A quality health and wellness store will carry better brands than what you'll find in other stores.

Intellect is a beautiful thing. Learning a new language is a great way to challenge yourself and connect with new people.

CILANTRO AND PARSLEY WATER

- 1 bunch cilantro
- 1 bunch parsley
- 8 cups of water

Cut into long pieces and put into a pot of boiling water. Cover and boil for one minute, then remove from heat. When the mixture is cold, strain and store it in a glass container in your refrigerator. Drink one glass of this water daily.

Benefits:

- Cleanses the body of toxins
- Cures kidney problems such as kidney stones, acting as a diuretic
- Stimulates liver functions
- Cures diarrhea
- Eliminates accumulated fat body
- Supports lowering cholesterol levels
- Heals mouth ulcers because it has antimicrobial and antiseptic properties
- Lowers blood sugars

• Helps with insomnia (without side effects of prescriptions!)

Note: Soaking your eyes with this water can help treat conjunctivitis.

APPLE CIDER VINEGAR

We've talked about how ACV is great for toning skin and promoting hair growth, but it also has a range of other benefits for overall wellness. In fact, it's been used for thousands of years around the world to treat all kinds of ailments. ACV can work wonders: it has antiseptic properties, can detoxify and flush the body, and treats illnesses and diseases.

You want raw, unfiltered vinegar (made from fermented apples), such as the kind made by Bragg. Drinking a mix of ACV and water can help with the following health conditions: arthritis, headaches, migraines, diarrhea, cough, sore throat, congestion, dizziness, vertigo, eczema, heartburn, bloody nose, insomnia, fatigue, food poisoning, high blood sugar, allergies and hay fever, hiccups, hearing problems, high cholesterol, inflammation, constipation, and obesity.

Although ACV is a powerful way to cure many health problems, use it with caution. This is especially true if you have diabetes or high blood pressure. You should research the recommended water-to-vinegar ratio for treating specific health issues (usually no stronger than 1 part vinegar per 5 parts water), and consult your doctor. Don't drink ACV straight; when consumed orally, the acidity can damage tooth enamel.

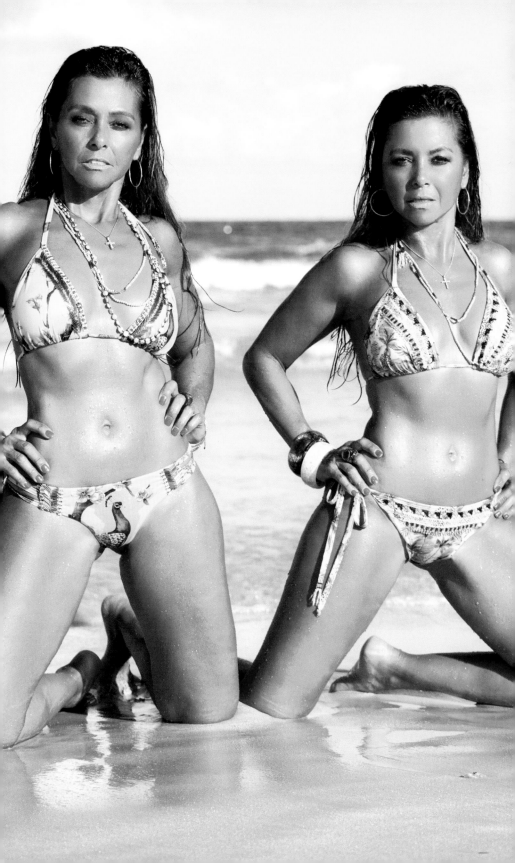

DAILY CLEANSE

- 1 teaspoon ACV
- 1 glass of filtered water
- A quarter of a lemon

Mix water and ACV, squeeze lemon into mixture, and drink. If you can't stand the taste of the ACV, add more water until you can stomach it. It might take a while to warm up to the idea of drinking vinegar water, but most people find it gets easier with practice.

Since ACV helps with so many health issues, we like to use it as an ongoing way to support wellness. It contains many important vitamins including B, C, biotin, folic acid, calcium, magnesium, anti-oxidants, and iron. This daily cleanse has many health benefits, such as enhancing digestion, diminishing inflammation, and providing natural alkalinity to balance stomach acids. But the main reason we drink it every single day is—drumroll please—WEIGHT LOSS! Don't get us wrong: ACV is not a substitution for going to the gym! But we have found that drinking a little ACV every day helps us maintain the low end of our weight range.

ACV DEODORANT

- 1 spoon of ACV
- 3 spoons of water
- 1 drop of lavender oil or tea tree oil

Apply the mixture with a cotton round. The ACV helps balance the pH of your skin. The antimicrobial properties in both the ACV and oils can reduce odor-causing bacteria.

Most antiperspirants have aluminum as the key ingredient, and there is much controversy over whether aluminum is linked to cancer. As with all products, it's best to err on the side of caution and go with something that definitely doesn't pose a health risk, such as a natural deodorant. It probably won't do as good of a job to keep you from sweating, but you'll still smell great.

COCONUT WATER

Coconut water has a range of health benefits you've probably never heard of. The most surprising fact is that it has a structure that is compatible with blood plasma in the human bloodstream. In wartime, when medical supplies were running short, coconut water was successfully used as an intravenous fluid in place of saline. Although most doctors today would never recommend a coconut water IV if there were other options, it is an all-natural and healthy beverage! Full of electrolytes and potassium, it's been proven to rehydrate the body better than water, helping to treat people who have diarrhea. Coconut water also detoxifies the body and acts as a natural diuretic, supporting kidney health. Rich in nutrients and anti-bacterial and anti-viral properties, it can strengthen your immune system and increase your energy. Last, it can help rev up your metabolism and promote weight loss. What more could you want?

Remember, you only get one body in this lifetime. You should treat it like your most valuable asset. If you aren't making your health and wellness a priority, now is the time to change!

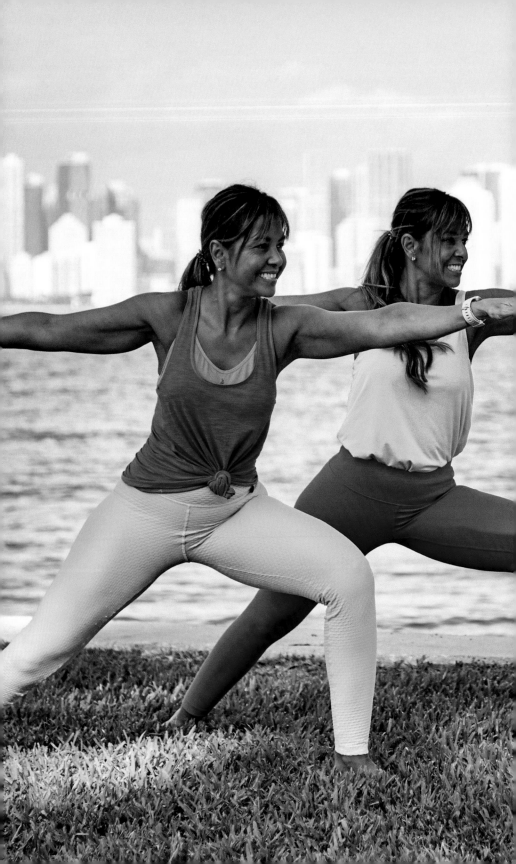

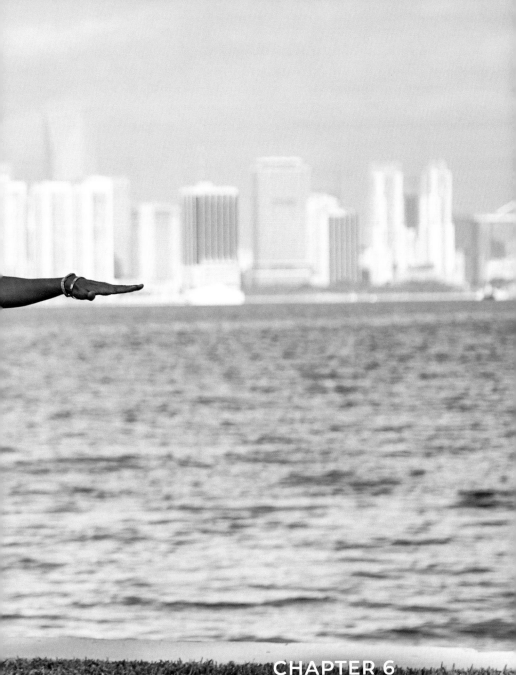

CHAPTER 6

Exercise

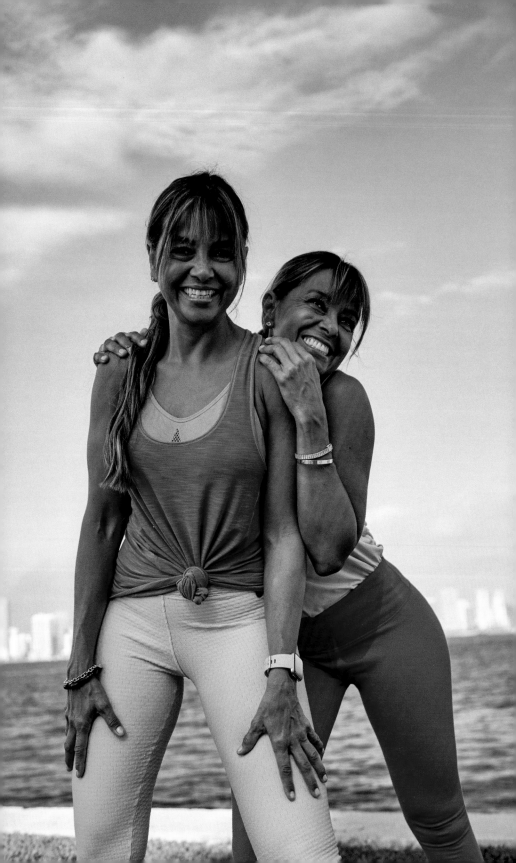

Exercise

Do you dream about having *the perfect* body? Most women do, but that vision can look totally different from person to person. We believe the perfect body is the one that makes you feel confident and proud. When you have those two feelings, you'll find that many things seem easier, from getting dressed in the morning, to speaking up in a meeting at work, to parting ways with people who don't treat you as well as they should.

Of course, you don't have to be physically fit to know your self-worth, but we've found that lack of fitness is something that often makes women feel badly about themselves. Feelings of unworthiness can derail life in a lot of ways. That's why it's so important for women to feel beautiful in their bodies. Some aspects of feeling beautiful come from a change in perspective, but sometimes it takes a physical change as well. That's why this chapter focuses on body positivity and making exercise easy.

Since we were young, we've made exercise a regular part of our lives. When we started modeling at age 12, we were advised to get a personal trainer to teach us how to exercise properly and stay fit. It might sound crazy that 12-year-olds had a personal trainer, but we loved it! We learned the proper form for lifting weights, what kind of exercises to do, and how those moves impact the body. Most importantly, we learned discipline for staying fit. Around the same age, we also started playing volleyball and doing spinning and aerobics, which were fun ways for us to be active. We exercised 4 to 6 times a week, and it felt great! Exercising as children made it easier to continue exercising into adulthood.

As long-time fitness models, we've had to embrace cardio and strength training as a major part of our lives. Even now, we work out almost every day because we love it. We're naturally athletic, and we really do enjoy working up a sweat. When we skip a workout, it almost feels like skipping a meal—like we're missing something essential!

We realize that a lot of people don't enjoy working out as much as we do, and that when you don't like something, it can be very hard to tap into your motivation to get it done. Working out can be more of a mental battle than a physical one. Since it takes mental strength to build good habits and force yourself to do things that are good for you, it helps to understand that there are also many mental benefits to exercise:

1. Creates clarity: For us, exercise brings clarity and focus to our lives. When we are struggling to make decisions about family, finances, or our careers, sometimes we feel like we're floundering or totally paralyzed. Exercise brings things into focus and makes decisions less stressful.

2. Improves energy: Although you might feel as if you're spending a lot of energy working out, studies show that regular exercise actually gives you more energy and boosts your vivacity to do things you love in life!

3. Reduces stress and balances hormones: You might not associate

stress with hormones levels, but guess what? Anxiety-induced hormonal fluctuations have negative effects on mood and energy levels. Being physically active helps you reduce stress and restore hormonal balance so that you feel like the best version of yourself.

4. Increases concentration: Exercise helps you develop the strength required to ignore those minor daily diversions and work toward what's really important. When we exercise regularly, we notice that we're more focused on our goals, regardless of distractions.

5. Promotes discipline: It is very important to make the time to work out, even with a busy, jam-packed schedule of work, family, and other personal commitments. When you exercise consistently, you become more disciplined in your life overall, making you a better employee, friend, and spouse.

Now that you know how great you'll feel by increasing your level of exercise, you need a plan for fitting it into your schedule. If you aren't a fitness model, you don't need to be working out every day unless you have the time for it and love it. Otherwise, exercising a few times a week might be enough for you.

In Spanish, we like to say, "*Matar ese pajaro temprano*," meaning you kill that bird in the morning by going to the gym as soon as you get up. Think about which exercises you enjoy the most and start with those at least three times a week until you get into the habit. Remember that power is in your mind, so you need to push yourself to do it. No pain, no gain.

Don't underestimate the power of music in staying young! Certain songs have a way of transforming your mood. Create the perfect workout playlist, and you might even forget you're exercising!

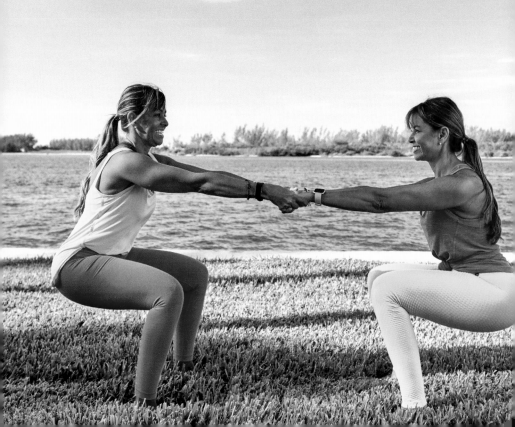

If you can afford personal training, we highly recommend it. You can work out with a friend to reduce the cost. We try to work out with a personal trainer twice a week because we learn different ways to keep our bodies in shape and ensure we have proper form so that we don't get injured. Trainers tailor workouts in ways that truly make a difference for getting the results we want.

When we work without a trainer, it's very easy to cruise slowly on the elliptical and do the same three or four other exercises, thinking it's making a difference. But it's really just taking up a lot of time and delivering little results. To make the most of a workout, you need to mix it up *a lot*. Doing so on your own is very difficult if you don't have a lot of health and fitness knowledge.

Group training classes have become very popular recently for this very reason, and we definitely recommend these classes, especially for people who are new to working out. When you do boot camp classes or high-intensity interval training (HIIT) classes, you do a variety of cardio and strength-training exercises in every class, and the exercises change from class to class. You can count on getting a great workout that will change your body shape and fitness level, and you don't have to do any planning or research. You just show up and work out.

Group classes are also great because they teach you different moves that you can do on your own later. More importantly, they show you what a good workout feels like. If you've been working out on your own at a gym and switch to group classes, you'll likely notice how much harder you're working out when someone is telling you what to do. Your heart rate goes higher, you lift heavier weights, and you're pushed more than you usually push yourself. That experience alone is valuable because it can help you set a new baseline for your workouts.

You should feel fantastic about yourself no matter how you look. Don't worry about what other people think. The only opinion that matters is your own. When you feel great about yourself, you will be better able to be there for your friends and family.

If the idea of working out harder doesn't sound that appealing, consider the benefits from a time perspective. Harder workouts don't take as long to get the same results. As you become fitter and can work out at a higher level, you can likely cut back the total time you spend in each workout session. For example, CrossFit is one of the most intense workouts. People compete doing a combination of prescribed exercises in as little time as possible. Some of the hardest workouts take seasoned athletes less than 10 minutes. You read that right—10 minutes! Don't get us wrong; they work out so hard in that time that they are completely exhausted, so it certainly isn't an easy option for exercise. But it shows that working out doesn't actually take as much time as people usually think.

When you know more about working out, you can make better choices to fit it into your life. For example, if you have only 20 or 30 minutes, you can do a good workout video at home without wasting any time commuting to a gym. If you don't have childcare when you want to work out, you can get a running stroller and run with your baby. Doing these kinds of shorter workouts several times a week will definitely make a difference.

We recommend trying a variety of exercises to see what you enjoy, and what seems to make the biggest difference in shaping the physique you want. Doing cardio almost every day helps us stay slim. Sometimes we do it on an empty stomach to burn more fat, and other times we do it after our weight training. Yes, we love lifting heavy weights! It really impacts not only building and toning our muscles, but burning fat as well. You might be totally different, and that's okay! We know women who hate lifting weights, but they swear by ballet-inspired barre workouts, hot yoga, Pilates, pole dancing, or many other types of exercises. Explore different workouts until you find options that you can do with energy, enthusiasm, and love.

You might be wondering how often you really need to be working out to get the results you want. The answer is a little different for everyone. If you live a very active lifestyle and eat healthy, you won't need as many workout sessions to stay fit as someone who has a sedentary lifestyle.

A lot of fit women and men live by one simple exercise rule: don't go more than three days without working out. (This rule stands even if you're on vacation or traveling for work.) It's great advice for a few reasons. The first is routine. People get into routines, and these routines can be hard to break. When you make exercise a routine, it isn't something you have to "feel like doing"; you just do it! The other reason is that your body burns more calories in the hours directly after exercise—called the afterburn effect. The number of extra calories burned and the amount of time they burn depend on how hard you work out, but your body will burn more calories on non-workout days that come directly after a workout day. For that reason, it's smart to space your workouts evenly throughout the week, rather than working out multiple days in a row and taking several days off. Burning more calories for the same amount of work is winning!

LIFE HACK TO REDUCE FAT AROUND YOUR WAIST

It's possible to target specific areas for weight loss while you work out. We recommend using an all-natural fat reduction or hot gel cream around your waist. The cream loosens fat tissue by temporarily dehydrating it, helping your metabolism make use of the fat as an energy source. After you apply the cream, cover it with osmotic body-wrap paper and put on an exercise belt. When you work out, you will sweat more around the waist, helping you lose water weight in that area. The

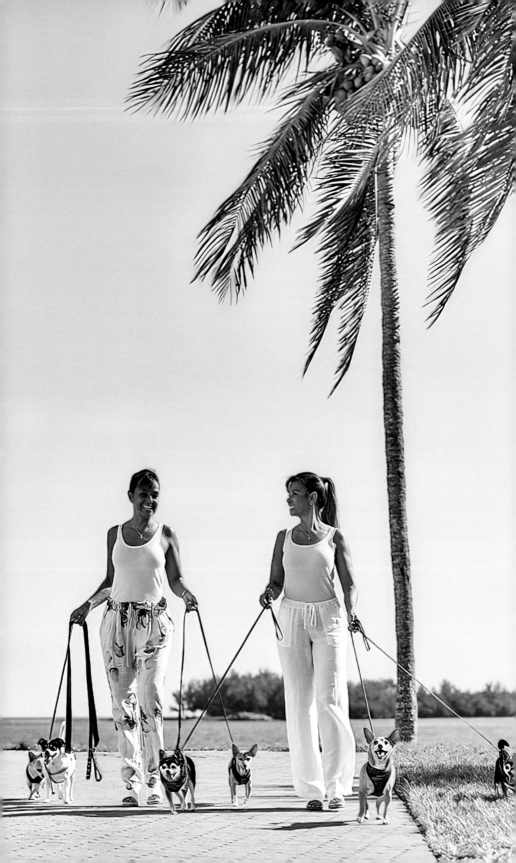

tightness of the band will also compress fat cells. These results combined can help you lose inches on your waist. The results are most dramatic right after you work out, so this beauty routine is especially great if you have an event or date night in the evening after your workout.

CONFIDENCE

No one can give you self-confidence. That has to come from within. You might think that when you look a certain way, you'll start to feel confident and sexy. While that might be true to a point, it's easy to keep finding little things that aren't perfect. If you focus on outward appearance, you won't ever be fully confident or happy with yourself. No matter what you look like today, now is the time to start feeling good about your body! As Latinas, this has always been very natural to us! We were raised to be proud of who we are and what we look like. As four-year-olds, we started wearing our mother's shoes and clothes, playing with her jewelry and makeup, and admiring ourselves in the mirror. We were so happy to do fashion shows for our parents, and they always made us feel beautiful. Years later, we still receive compliments from family and friends for the way we were brought up—to feel valued and confident.

Your self-esteem is your engine, and your confidence is the transmission that puts it into motion. As twins, we have always been each other's biggest supporters. We don't cut each other down or begrudge each other's successes. We build each other up, and we're each other's biggest cheerleaders. Having that kind of emotional support has impacted our self-esteem over the years.

Learn to love your body, respecting and accepting it the way it is. Stop being so demanding about changing yourself! Release the prejudices you hold about your figure (e.g., too big, too small, etc.) These viewpoints distract you from what really matters in life.

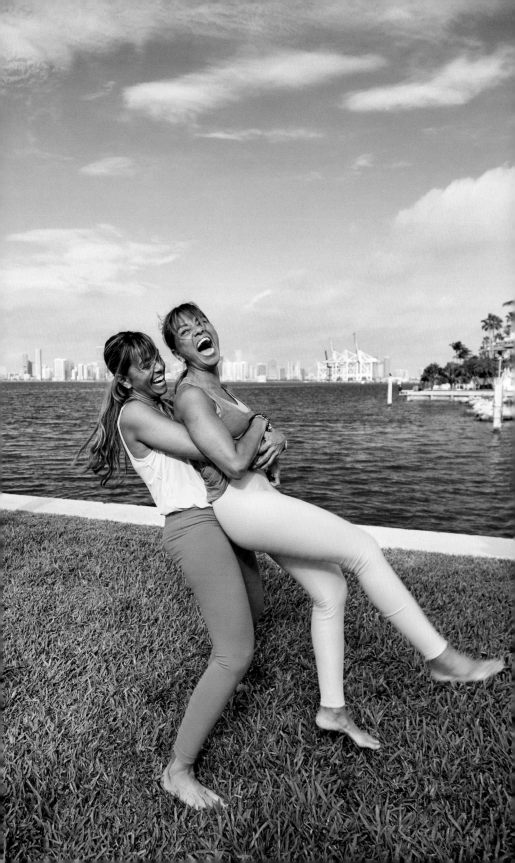

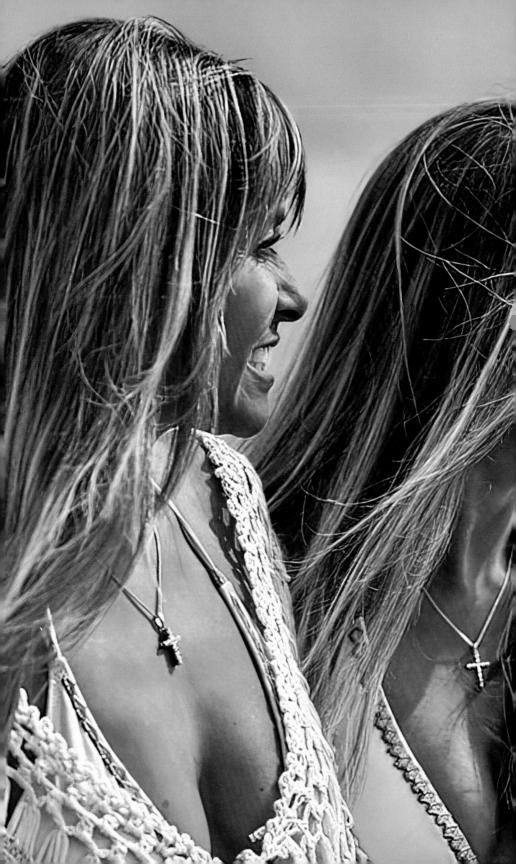

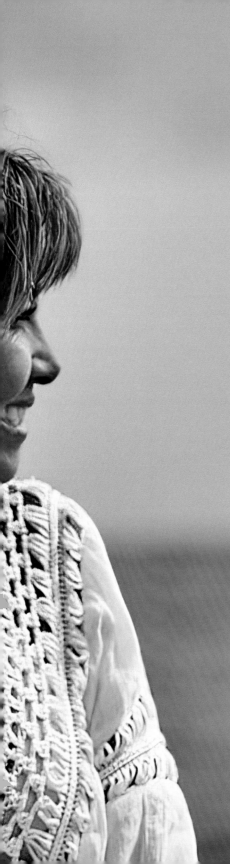

CHAPTER 7

Breasts

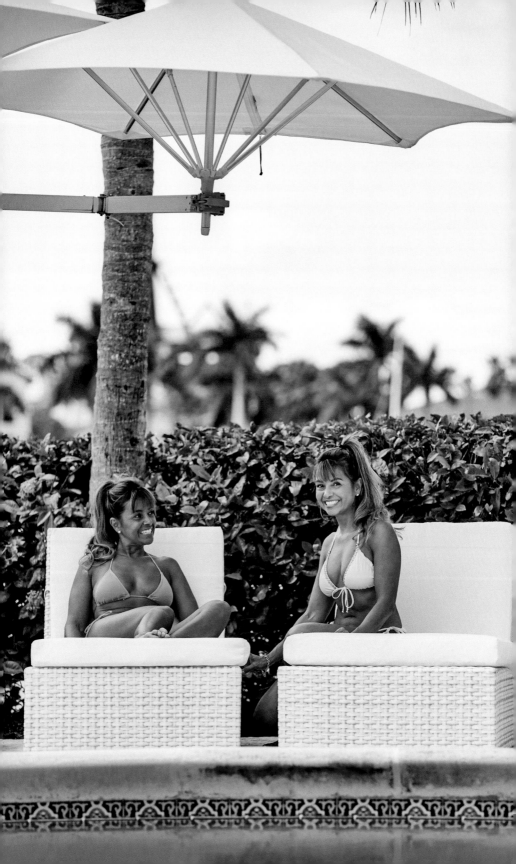

Breasts

Breasts are sensual. No matter their size or shape, they are a symbol of our femininity. We remember seeing our breasts first emerge in college, and it was a strange feeling. It seemed special—a unique power that only women hold.

While we can't do much to change our genetic makeup, we can take better care of our assets—particularly making them stay perky, full, and firm. Here are our best secrets for having naturally beautiful breasts.

MAINTAINING ELASTICITY

Genetics play a factor in perkiness, but lifestyle is even more important. The goal is to keep elasticity in the skin on your breasts to prevent stretching and sagging. Of course, stretching and sagging are unavoidable over time, but you can keep your breasts looking younger longer with the following tips.

AVOID WEIGHT FLUCTUATION

When you gain weight, you gain it all over your body, including your breasts. When you lose that weight, your fat disappears, but your extra skin doesn't. Unless you're gaining and losing a great deal of weight, skin that's a little looser isn't usually that noticeable—except in your breasts. Gravity starts pulling your breasts south from the time they first sprout on your chest, and extra skin does not help the situation. Maintaining a healthy diet and exercise routine will help keep your breasts looking younger longer.

DON'T SQUEEZE OR STRETCH

You want to be as gentle as possible with your breasts. Make sure you give them support from a good bra, especially if you have large, heavy breasts. When your breasts hang, the weight pulls your skin. The same thing happens when you work out without a good sports bra—the bouncing stretches your skin. Also beware of bras that are too tight because they can squeeze the breasts, stretching the skin by flattening it down. Lying on your stomach can have the same skin-stretching effect.

TRY HYDROTHERAPY

Water temperature can impact the skin's elasticity. When we were young, we learned to splash our breasts with cold water after a warm a bath or shower to help the skin stay firm. We also sometimes put ice on our breasts, which not only feels great on a hot day, but helps tone the skin. It might sound crazy, but there's science behind what seems like an old wives' tale for beautiful breasts. Alternating from hot to cold temperature improves blood circulation, which stimulates the

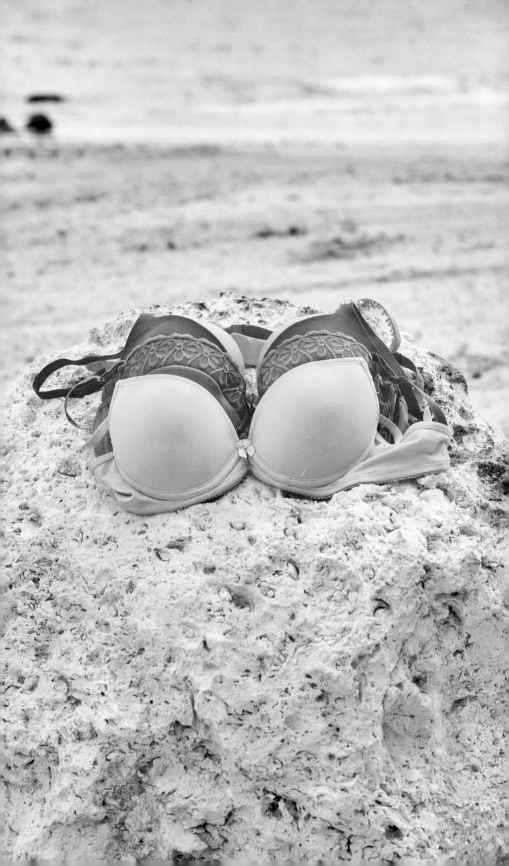

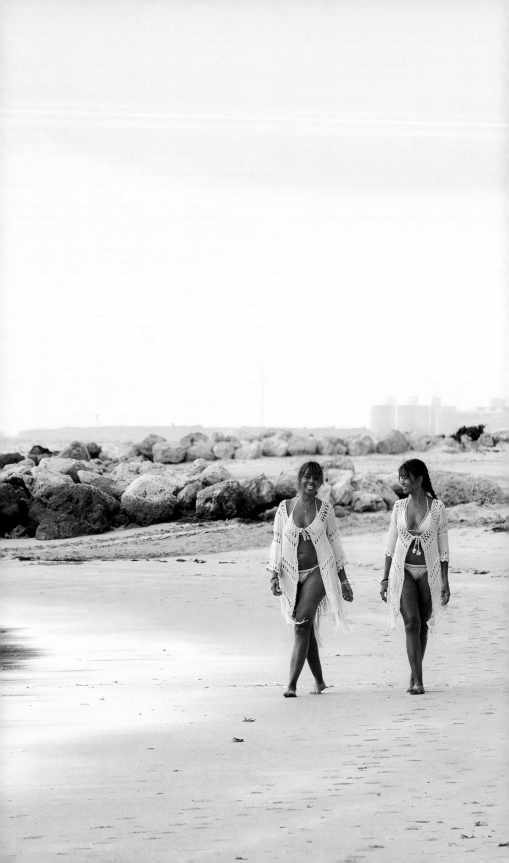

production of collagen and elastin, increasing skin's firmness. Blood circulation can also stimulate the growth of local tissues, helping improve fullness. We've known women who have kept their breasts full and perky after having multiple children, and they swear by giving their breasts ice water baths in their bathroom sink.

IMPROVE YOUR POSTURE

When you have poor posture, your shoulders bend forward, and your breasts have less support against gravity, especially when you're not wearing a bra. It also gives the appearance that your breasts are hanging lower, in a less desirable shape. Your mother was right—it is important to sit and stand up straight!

WORK YOUR MUSCLES

Many exercises tone the muscles behind and around your breasts. Toning these muscles can make your breasts look higher and firmer. Try exercises like pushups, planks, and the dumbbell fly.

PROTECT AGAINST THE SUN

The skin on your chest is especially sensitive. Easily burned, it is prone to wrinkling more than other parts of the body. Vertical wrinkles in the cleavage area can become more prominent (and higher on the chest) than cleavage—something you want to avoid! Protect against the sun's harmful rays with sunscreen, and stay out of the sun in the middle of the day when the sun is the strongest. It's also smart to avoid black bras and swimsuits, because they absorb more sunlight directly than other colors and can increase your risk of breast cancer.

BREAST HEALTH

According to the National Cancer Institute, 1 in 8 women will get breast cancer at some point in her life. We all need to think about reducing our risk and preparing to catch it early just in case it happens.

- Check your breasts for lumps. Poke gently with the pads of your fingers. Start from the outside of your breasts and work in a circular motion toward the nipples to feel your entire breast. If anything feels unusual, make a doctor's appointment immediately.
- Get yearly mammograms once you turn 40. If you have a family history of breast cancer, talk to your doctor about getting mammograms when you're younger.
- Eat organic. It is a sad truth that there are known cancer-causing chemicals in foods that are legally sold to us. Reduce your exposure to these chemicals and carcinogens by eating organic whenever possible.

EGG WHITE MASK

- 1 fresh egg white

Apply gently to your breasts and chest. Let dry for 15 minutes and wash off with soap and water.

This mask works like a face lift for your breasts. You'll notice tighter skin that appears firmer. Apply mask before you take a shower.

TIPS FOR BEAUTIFUL BREASTS

- Blood circulation can help your body grow tissue. For women, more tissue means fuller breasts. Olive oil has many nutrients that promote blood circulation, so we recommend massaging it onto the breasts in a circular motion. Oil is good for the skin, so you wouldn't need to rinse or wash it off. Another great option is to use a soft brush to massage your breasts and activate the blood circulation.
- You can exfoliate your breasts gently with a body scrub, and then moisturize them with sweet almond oil. This oil is a powerful antioxidant, helping your skin maintain its collagen level.

With breast augmentation surgery becoming quite common, more and more women feel like they don't measure up. We're here to tell you that you don't need surgery to look and feel beautiful! Surgery is always a risk, and putting anything unnatural inside your body for the sake of beauty is silly. If you want to improve the appearance of your breasts, all you have to do is take care of them. We've been doing the things in this chapter for years, and we feel great about ours, even as we get older. Having firm, perky breasts makes us feel elegant and feminine, and we know you'll feel the same way by trying our natural beauty secrets for yourself.

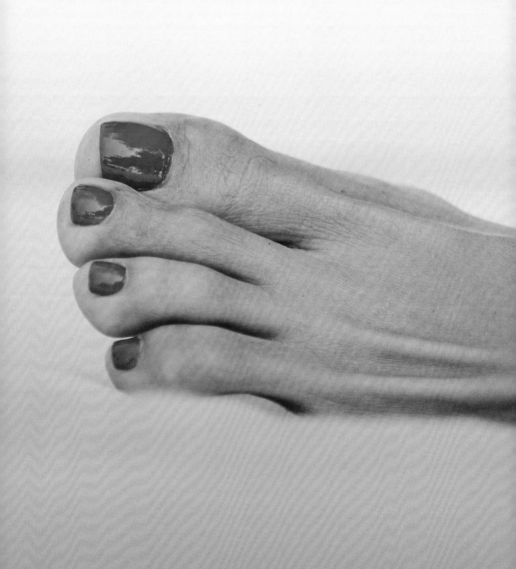

CHAPTER 8

Feet

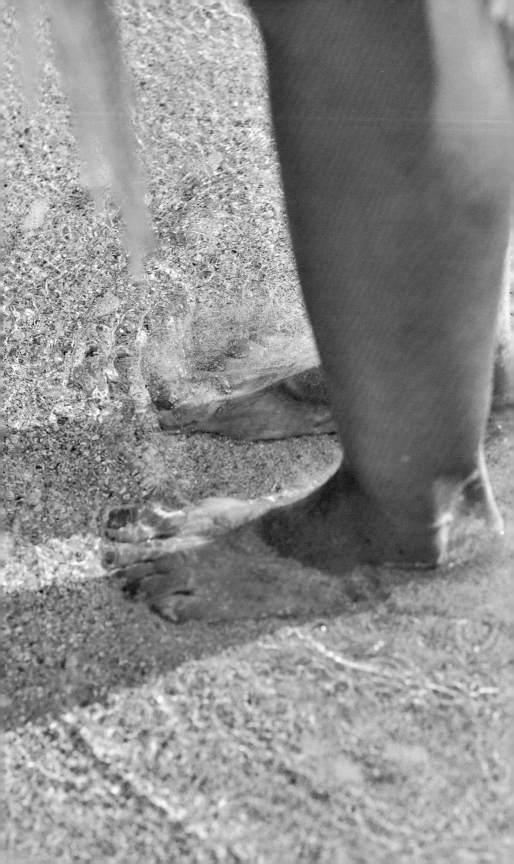

Feet

When you think about beauty, feet might not be the first thing to come to mind. But you use your feet all day long, and you rely on them for living your best life. Given how much work they do and how much weight they carry, you should be nice to your feet!

Calluses, rough skin, and unhealthy nails are common issues that cause women to feel insecure about their feet. Because we live in Miami, our feet are exposed to many damaging elements. Since the weather is always right for sandals and open-toe shoes, we don't get a chance to hide them! Here are our best tips for keeping feet healthy and beautiful.

FIND THE RIGHT SHOES

Your feet are the most beautiful when they do what they are meant to do—get you to where you want to go without pain! That's why beauty for this chapter starts with function. Don't underestimate the importance of wearing good shoes.

HEELS

High heels are sexy, but they can cause long-term damage to your feet if you wear them too much. Being in the world of modeling, we know many women who have a lot of foot pain from spending too much time in heels. You might think the pain is temporary and will end when you take off your heels, but that isn't always the case. Wearing heels puts a lot more pressure on the balls of your feet, and it can actually wear down the fat pads that provide natural cushioning, leading to long-term pain. Extra weight on the front of your feet can also cause pinched nerves and stress fractures. We know a model who worked a job that required walking in stilettos all day for several days in a row. Her feet hurt very badly, but she kept going because it was her job. After that, three of her toes went numb for several weeks, and her foot swelled so much that it wouldn't fit in any of her shoes. She went to a podiatrist, and you know what he told her? Stop wearing heels. You may think heels are sexy and glamorous, but they are not meant to be worn day in and day out. When you buy heels, go for options that have a little more cushioning and support, such as a wedge or a thicker heel.

WORKOUT SHOES

Since staying fit and active is an essential part of living a healthy life, you need good workout shoes. Most women choose workout shoes based on how they look, but that's the wrong approach. Workout shoes are made for different purposes and different types of feet. Getting the right pair will make your workouts more enjoyable and help you avoid injuries.

If you plan on going running, which is one of the most accessible ways to stay fit, find a shoe store where an expert can watch you run and advise you and suggest the right kind of shoe to buy. The expert will video you running on a treadmill and then watch the video in slow-motion to spot any issues to watch out for, such as over or under-pronating, which is when your ankles naturally roll in or out a bit more than they should. Based on how you run, you'll get a recommendation on the level of support you should have in your shoes (e.g., a stability shoe or a natural shoe). You can also get insoles for an even better fit. This kind of help can totally change your experience as a runner. Good shoes change the way your whole body moves when you run. You can go from struggling to run a mile to working up to a 5K, 10K, or even a marathon!

FOOT SOAK

- A half cup of sea salt
- About a gallon and a half of water
- 5 to 10 drops of essential oil
  - Lavender oil has calming effects, such as slowing the activity in the central nervous system.
  - Tea tree oil is antimicrobial and antifungal.
  - Blue chamomile oil is anti-inflammatory (perfect for swollen feet), and the aroma produces a mild sedative effect that makes you sleepy.

Add ingredients to a foot bath and soak your feet for about 10 minutes. Sea salt is a great source of minerals to alkalize the body, and it helps reduce stress and foot odors. Don't leave your feet too long in the water because salt has a drying effect that will ultimately leave your feet dry and cracked.

NAILS

We always keep our toenails trimmed, cutting them about twice a month. We're careful not to cut nails too short—they should be about the same length as the toes. We cut the nail straight across rather than rounding the edges. Not only does that create a pleasing look, it helps prevent ingrown toenails. (Ingrown nails are not fun! They cause your toes to swell and make walking painful. You definitely want to avoid them!) We skip the cuticle-cutting on our feet, even when getting a pedicure. Cuticles protect toes from infection, so we don't do anything to get rid of them.

We usually have polish on our toes, but polish can take a toll on nails. Try to use polish that doesn't contain harmful chemicals like formaldehyde. When you switch to a better polish, you'll probably notice healthier nails, and longer-lasting pedicures. That said, it's always good to take a break from polish occasionally to give your toenails a breather and allow them to regain moisture. A couple of weeks or a month off is usually enough time to rejuvenate nails.

Even good nail polish can stain. If you have yellowing on your nails, you can scrub them with lemon juice or baking soda and water to help get rid of surface stains. You can also gently buff off stains with an emery board.

ACV SOAK FOR TREATING NAIL FUNGUS

- 1 cup ACV
- 2 cups water

Add ingredients to a foot bath and soak your feet for about 15 minutes. Do this regularly until your nails heal. (For bad cases, this is not a substitute for medicine.)

TIPS FOR BEAUTIFUL FEET

- Exfoliating is important for removing dead skin cells and keeping feet smooth and soft. You can use a salt or sugar scrub.
- Use a pumice stone on the bottoms of your feet to buff off calluses.
- A lot of oils that act as natural moisturizers are lost through day-to-day walking, so you should moisturize your feet on a regular basis. At bedtime, rub Vaseline, coconut oil, or pure shea butter on your feet and put on a pair of socks right after. You will see the difference in the morning.
- To help extend your pedicure, try applying a new layer of topcoat every 2 days or so to protect against chips and nicks.

Recognize when you're having negative thoughts. Do everything you can to transform your outlook and feel positive.

Every night before bedtime, write down your achievements for that day. Think about how tomorrow will be an even better day.

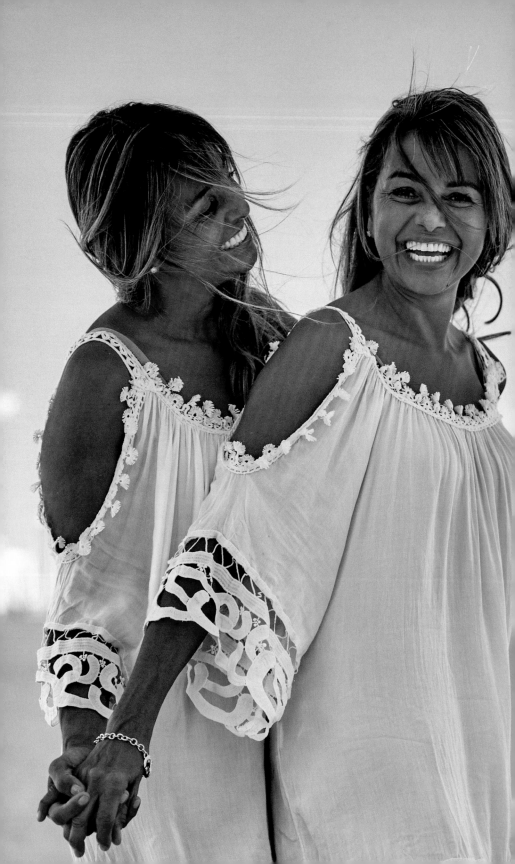

CHAPTER 9

Aging Gracefully

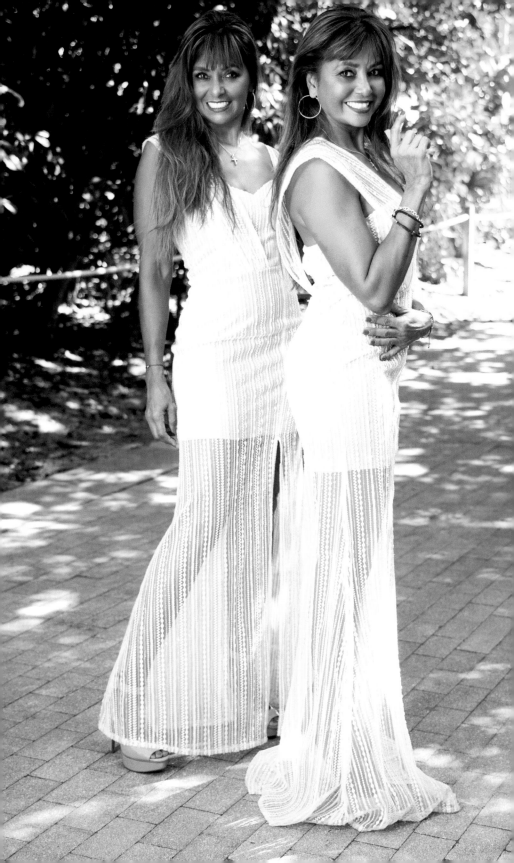

Aging Gracefully

Don't be afraid of getting older. We all get older, and it beats the alternative! Our father always tells us that there are three ages:

- The one you really have
- The one you represent
- The one that people give to you

We don't want to just look young—we want to feel young. That feeling comes from being healthy and having a positive outlook. We meet people all the time who think we're in our early 20s! (And this is even when we aren't wearing makeup!) They call us "girls" and ask how we look so young. We tell them we have been taking care of ourselves from a very young age. It sounds like a simple answer, but it's the truth.

This book is the result of more than 35 years of constant dedication to the secrets of beauty and health. If you follow the advice in this book with discipline and consistency, you will see a dramatic difference in your face, neck, teeth, hair, skin, breasts, feet, and your whole body. And when you take care of your whole body, you will not only see a physical change, you will feel the difference in your mind and spirit.

Self-care enables us to be our best selves. When we are healthy, well-rested, well-nourished, and feeling good about living in our body, we are in a much better spot to live our purpose and make an impact in the world. The secrets in this book will help you look twenty years younger and more beautiful, but your physical appearance will never compare to the beauty that's inside.

We are happy to say we prioritize love. Love is the most powerful emotion a human being can experience, so we work to fill our hearts with it. We prioritize each other, our family members, our close friends, and our pets. (Together, we own six chihuahuas!) We do the best we can to be there for the people and animals we love, spending quality time with them whenever possible.

We also prioritize love in our work. Our home country of Venezuela has been going through tough times. Growing up, we lived a beautiful life. But now the supermarket shelves are empty, hospitals don't have medicine, and people don't have access to basic necessities like toilet paper. If fact, so many Venezuelans are starving that people are getting desperate to feed their families, and it's become incredibly dangerous. With 35,000 murders a year, the country is essentially a war zone. People are afraid to leave their homes after dark for fear of being killed for the shoes on their feet.

This reality has absolutely broken our hearts. We are safe living in the United States, but we couldn't sleep at night thinking of our family, friends, and everyone else back home suffering. So we created a family foundation to help, called Fundación Solidarios con Venezuela. We deliver food, medicine, and supplies to people and animals in need within the Andes region. The U.S. chapter is based out of Miami, and we collect new and used donations from the community on an ongoing basis. Every month, we send boxes to the people of Venezuela, including clothes, shoes, blankets, toiletries, and over-the-counter medicine.

We never imagined the work of our family being able to reach so many people, and we thank God for the impact we have been able to make. Every month, our foundation provides meals for children in three different schools so that they don't go hungry. We also provide hospitals with the equipment to help save premature babies. And every month, we support 350 stray dogs, providing food, toys, and vaccines. We are excited to donate a portion of all book sales to Fundación Solidarios con Venezuela. Helping people fulfills us in a way that nothing else does. We believe that being disciplined in taking care of ourselves has made it easier for us to take care of others.

We hope this book inspires you to take the action you need to improve your life in a meaningful way, whether by eating better, exercising more, soaking your feet, or ultimately reshaping your life to follow your dreams. We want you to know that you are beautiful and worthy of everything great in the world.

Relationships don't thrive on auto-pilot. Make time for the people you care about, and don't forget to cultivate new friendships. You have to give mucho amor to receive love back.

Remember that time is one of the most precious resources we have. Once it is gone, we can never get it back. By living a healthier, happier life, you can actually add more years onto your life! We ask you to make a pledge to start living your best life today. Not tomorrow—*today.*

> Love like you haven't been hurt. You get the most out of relationships when you really dive into them.

Here are some suggestions to get started:

- Try a new recipe in this book that caught your eye.
- Plan a fun new workout.
- Make a healthy meal with ingredients you love.
- Call an old friend.
- Tell your family members you love them.
- Go to bed early tonight.
- Look in the mirror and tell yourself you're beautiful just as you are.
- Think about how you can do something positive to help others.

Time goes by so fast. Before we know it, we'll be little old ladies! Let's enjoy life as it comes and make the most out of it!

Sincerely,

Marita and Mimina Meza

As we get older, it's important to continue focusing on self-development. Physical beauty might peak at a younger age, but what's inside keeps getting better. The older you get, the better you know yourself. You're able to make better, wiser decisions about your life and what makes you happy. You can refocus your attention on what really matters, like being a good person and helping others.

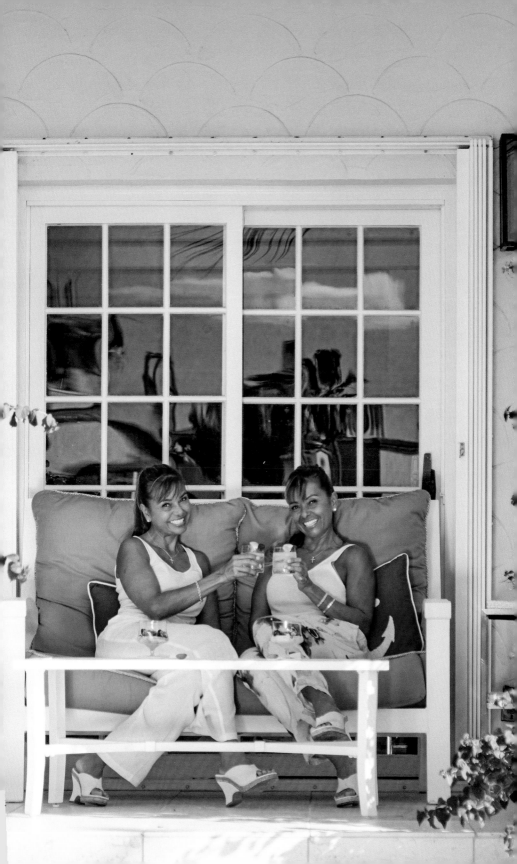

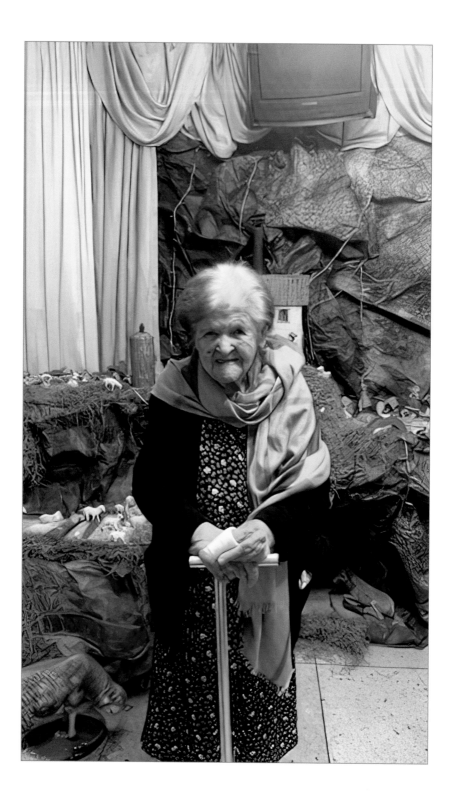

ACKNOWLEDGMENTS

SPECIAL THANKS TO Dan Gerstein from Gotham Ghostwriters, who, with his knowledge, experience, and faith in our book, guided us to the right people and helped one of our dreams come true: this amazing book!

To Jesus our Lord. No matter where we are or what challenges we face, God is always in control of our lives. He's always directing our steps, and He has us exactly where he wants us to be.

To Jonathan Holtz, for the brilliant idea to write this book. Your expertise and guidance have been invaluable. We love you.

To Adriana Gómez, our personal trainer, for making us work hard on our bodies, and for teaching us the best exercises to stay in shape.

To our editor, Amelia Forczak, for your belief and faith in us, and for pushing us with your hard work.

To both of our photographers, John Olive and Julian Retrepo, for the amazing pictures. Thank you to both of you for investing your energy in this project.

To Mireya Meza, our younger sister. Your talented hands made this book, and our natural look, possible. Our makeup was always perfect and impeccable!

To our loyal sister, Yudith Meza Vergara, for being our "third triplet" It was not easy for you to handle double trouble, and you were always there in good times and in bad.

To all our family and friends, for the enthusiasm and energy you gave us to finish and publish this book.

To Tia Panchita Vergara, our aunt who just turned 103 years old and graciously took the time to share with us many of the natural beauty secrets that changed our lives.

Thank you to all our little furry ones. There is nothing more beautiful in this world than their unconditional love.

Most of all, to our parents, Aminta Vergara Noguera and Napoleon Meza Febres, who gave us the best education, love, and support, and who guided us from day one.

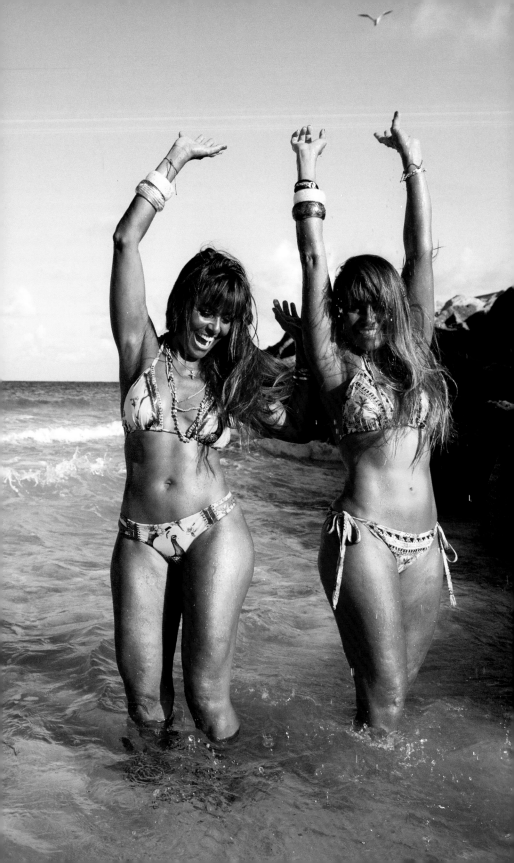